MRCPsych

PART I
PRACTICE PAPERS:
ISQs AND EMIs

To James

MRCPsych

PART I
PRACTICE PAPERS:
ISQs AND EMIs

NICHOLAS TAYLOR
MB ChB MRCPsych

Specialist Registrar in Forensic Psychiatry
Reaside Clinic, Birmingham

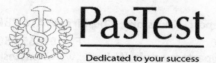

PasTest

Dedicated to your success

© 2005 PasTest Ltd
Egerton Court
Parkgate Estate
Knutsford
Cheshire, WA16 8DX

Telephone: 01565 752000

First edition 2005

ISBN: 1 904 627 595

A catalogue record for this book is available from the British Library.

The information contained within this book was obtained by the
author from reliable sources. However, while every effort has been
made to ensure its accuracy, no responsibility for loss, damage or
injury occasioned to any person acting or refraining from action as a
result of information contained herein can be accepted by the
publisher or the author.

PasTest Revision Books and Intensive Courses

PasTest has been established in the field of postgraduate medical
education since 1972, providing revision books and intensive study
courses for doctors preparing for their professional examinations.
Books and courses are available for the following specialties:

MRCP Part 1 and Part 2, MRCPCH Part 1 and Part 2, MRCOG,
DRCOG, MRCGP, MRCPsych, DCH, FRCA, MRCS and PLAB.

For further details contact:

PasTest Ltd, Freepost, Knutsford, Cheshire, WA16 7BR
Tel: **01565 752000**   Fax: **01565 650264**
Email: **enquiries@pastest.co.uk** Web site: **www. pastest.co.uk**

Typeset by The Old Tin Dog Design Company, Brighton, UK
Printed and bound by MPG Ltd, Bodmin, UK

CONTENTS

CONTENTS

INTRODUCTION

The aim of this book is to help you to prepare for the MRCPsych Part I ISQs and EMIs. There are several practice questions available for this exam, but many are out of date, inaccurate or simply wrong. The questions and answers in this book are modelled as closely as possible on the current exam. The format is exactly the same and there is a close correlation between the subject areas covered in this book and those covered in the real exam.

Almost every question has an explanation and a cross-reference for further information. By flicking through this book, you will be able to revise many different areas very quickly and by practising papers against time limits just before the exam you will be able to make sure that you are able to keep to the tight time limits of the real exam. The answers are referenced, where relevant, to other textbooks in the PasTest range: *Essential Revision Notes in Psychiatry for MRCPsych* edited by Christopher Fear, *The A-Z of the MRCPsych* by Nicholas Taylor and *A Guide to Psychiatric Examination* by Carmelo Aquilina and James Warner.

EMIs are a source of anxiety for exam candidates as the format is relatively new and there are not as many practice questions available. The 60 EMIs in this book cover all the common areas tested in the real exam and are perfect preparation. It is important to remember that the EMIs account for a disproportionate number of marks. Each EMI 'theme' has three individual questions or 'stems'. Each of these 'stems' is worth three marks, so the EMI section accounts for 90 marks out of a total of 223 marks – almost half of the total.

Preparation is the key to passing the Part I and this book will help you to prepare. You will then be less likely to face the difficult job of revising for a second time.

EXAMINATION TECHNIQUE

Passing the Part I depends on adequate revision and preparation. Although there is an element of luck in every exam, you will not pass without the knowledge. Many candidates try to prepare for the exam by reading textbooks in the hope that they can learn enough to pass. This seems a sensible way to proceed, but the exam tends to test knowledge about particular areas of the syllabus time and time again, leaving out large chunks completely. Revision from textbooks is important, but revising by looking at practice questions is often more productive.

This book will help you to revise most productively because the questions and answers within it are based closely on the questions in the real exam. This means that the most important parts of the syllabus are covered comprehensively and the areas which are rarely tested are given less attention.

This book can be used in several ways. Flick through it and you will find you can answer some of the questions, even before you have started revising. Other questions will highlight areas which you know almost nothing about – these can then be revised more thoroughly. Save some of the practice papers for the last few weeks before the exam and then try to answer them within the tight time limit (90 minutes per paper) of the real exam. You will be surprised at how little time is allowed, but it is better to realise this 2 weeks before the exam than on the day itself.

On the day of the exam, answer all the questions you are sure about and which you can answer quickly. Leave the questions you are stuck on – you do not have time to sit and think about them for more than just a few seconds. Move on, answer the other questions and come back to the difficult questions at the end. There is no negative marking so you must answer every question, even if some answers are little more than guesses.

Extended matching items (EMIs) are new to many candidates and they account for a disproportionately high number of marks, with every answer to an EMI stem accounting for three marks, compared with one mark for an answer to an individual statement question (ISQ). The format of the EMIs is confusing at first and practising these is particularly important.

Preparation for the exam is fundamental to success, and this book is one of the most effective ways of preparing. I hope you find it as helpful as others have in passing the Part 1.

Nicholas Taylor

PRACTICE PAPER 1

Time allowed: 90 minutes

INDIVIDUAL STATEMENT QUESTIONS

1.1   Risperidone is a dibenzazepine.

1.2   Alzheimer's disease has equal sex incidence.

1.3   Motivation can be explained in terms of homeostatic mechanisms.

1.4   Couvade syndrome is very rare.

1.5   First-pass metabolism is increased with intravenous rather than intramuscular administration.

1.6   The ego contains primordial energy from instinctual drives.

1.7   Cognitive assessment involves assessment of the level of consciousness.

1.8   The dose equivalent of clozapine 50 mg is chlorpromazine 100 mg.

1.9   Akathisia can be difficult to distinguish from tardive dyskinesia.

1.10   Common symptoms of couvade syndrome include nausea and fatigue.

1.11   Figure–ground discrimination refers exclusively to the ability to perceive a person against a dark background.

1.12   Monoamine oxidase inhibitors should not be used in conjunction with opiates.

1.13   Fear is entirely unconscious.

1.14 Citalopram has marked effects on the cytochrome p450 enzyme system.

1.15 Falls are more common in Alzheimer's disease than in Lewy body dementia.

1.16 Smoked herrings are safe to eat in conjunction with monoamine oxidase inhibitors.

1.17 The phenomenon of approximate answers is also known as *vorbeireden*.

1.18 Attitudes are determined by conative, affective and behavioural components.

1.19 Dreams are composed of the night residue and nocturnal stimuli.

1.20 Attitude discrepant behaviour is rare in humans.

1.21 The establishment of identity and avoidance of confusion is an important process which Erikson identified in adolescents.

1.22 Bowlby proposed affectionless psychopathy as a consequence of deprivation of attachment.

1.23 De Clerambault's syndrome is usually seen in married women.

1.24 Jung described dreams as 'the royal road to the unconscious'.

1.25 It is inappropriate to discuss suicidal ideation in the first interview, as this is too upsetting.

1.26 Declarative memory concerns motor skills.

1.27 Groups are more likely than individuals to reach extreme conclusions.

1.28 Hallucinations are voluntary.

1.29 Encoding, storage and retrieval must all be intact for memory to function effectively.

1.30   Alexia is the inability to recognise one's own emotions.

1.31   Atypical antipsychotics are always preferable to typical antipsychotics.

1.32   Denial is a sophisticated defence mechanism.

1.33   Absorption of diazepam after intramuscular administration is significantly reduced by binding of the drug within the tissue.

1.34   Avocados contain tyramine.

1.35   Somatic passivity and made actions are first-rank symptoms of schizophrenia.

1.36   *Vorbeigehen* is a feature of Ganser's syndrome.

1.37   Late paraphrenia is distinguished from other types of paraphrenia in the International Statistical Classification of Diseases and Related Health Problems, 10th revision (ICD-10).

1.38   Foucault and Klein were prominent anti-psychiatrists.

1.39   Chunking can allow more effective use of available memory.

1.40   γ-Amino butyric acid (GABA)-A receptors have both GABA and flumazenil as agonists.

1.41   Clang associations are more suggestive of schizophrenia than of mania.

1.42   Depression occurring after cerebrovascular accident results from neurological rather than social factors in most cases.

1.43   Thurstone's scale measures processing speed.

1.44   Distractibility is increased in mania.

1.45   Tyrosine is involved in the synthetic chain of dopamine production.

1.46 Piaget's preoperational stage lasts from approximately 7 to 12 years.

1.47 It is inappropriate to ask patients about suicide because it may prompt them to commit suicide, even if the patient had not considered it previously.

1.48 Learned helplessness can only be observed in dogs.

1.49 The double jeopardy hypothesis suggests that older people engage more actively in society because they have nothing to lose.

1.50 Chronic high-dose use of a typical antipsychotic can cause discoloration of the conjunctiva, retina and cornea.

1.51 Coma is also known as the coenestopathic state.

1.52 Formication may be experienced during alcohol withdrawal.

1.53 The cheese reaction can also be precipitated by cream cheese.

1.54 Derailment is a breakdown in connections within thoughts.

1.55 Lysergic acid diethylamide is a 5-hydroxytryptamine (5HT) agonist.

1.56 The physical symptoms experienced in Ganser's syndrome are a result of somatisation.

1.57 The International Statistical Classification of Diseases and Related Health Problems, 10th revision (ICD-10) classification system is only available in one version.

1.58 The Schneiderian symptoms of schizophrenia were described by Carl Schneider.

1.59 Postural hypotension and ejaculatory failure result from the antihistaminergic actions of typical antipsychotics.

1.60 Eidetic imagery is common among children.

1.61 The central antimuscarinic effects of typical antipsychotics lead to pyrexia and a dry mouth.

1.62 Pyrexia has been reported as a cause of manic states.

1.63 In preparation for an interview, two chairs should be positioned so that they face each other directly. This enables proper assessment of eye contact during the interview.

1.64 A change in one of the components of an attitude does not change the attitude itself, as the other two components remain constant in most cases.

1.65 Schizophrenic hallucinations are typically very well localised in space.

1.66 Believing it to be five past three rather than five to three indicates significant disorientation in time.

1.67 Anxiety usually includes a subjective sense of constriction.

1.68 Behavioural and emotional problems are more common in families with only one parent.

1.69 More than 95% of an oral dose of lithium is subsequently excreted in the urine.

1.70 The Diagnostic and Statistical Manual of Mental Disorders-IV (DSM-IV) includes a broader definition of schizophrenia than International Statistical Classification of Diseases and Related Health Problems, 10th revision (ICD-10).

1.71 Tricyclic antidepressants are hydrophilic.

1.72 Clozapine is associated with sialorrhoea.

1.73 Typical antipsychotics antagonise dopamine, acetylcholine, adrenaline and histamine receptors.

1.74 Antagonism of autoreceptors can result in increased neurotransmission.

1.75 Dopamine has a direct stimulating effect on adrenergic receptors.

1.76 Illusions are a form of hallucination.

1.77 Thought stopping is also known as thought sonalisation.

1.78 The id is mostly conscious.

1.79 More effort has to be made to retrieve information from short-term memory than from long-term memory.

1.80 Kurt Schneider described fusion, derailment and omission.

1.81 During a progressive dementing process, individuals characteristically become disoriented in place before they become disoriented in time.

1.82 Forgetting usually results from failure of retrieval from memory.

1.83 Extracampine hallucinations are usually olfactory in nature.

1.84 Bromocriptine is a dopamine receptor antagonist.

1.85 The first- and second-rank symptoms of schizophrenia were described by Carl Schneider.

1.86 Thorndike and Skinner were both important in the development of the theory of operant conditioning.

1.87 Affect is synonymous with mood.

1.88 The mere exposure effect causes one to dislike people from different backgrounds whenever one encounters them.

1.89 Disorientation in time occurs before disorientation in place or person.

1.90   Inverse agonists are also known as antagonists.

1.91   Clozapine is the only antipsychotic that does not cause the neuroleptic malignant syndrome.

1.92   Freud believed that dreams indicated conflict between the id and the ego.

1.93   Within a family, younger children are more likely to refuse school than older children.

1.94   Phenothiazine antipsychotics cause weight gain with no associated increase in appetite.

1.95   Corticosteroid use can precipitate both depressive and manic states.

1.96   Hallucinations are misperceptions of external stimuli.

1.97   Stimulus preparedness explains why more people are afraid of spiders than of cats.

1.98   Behaviours with survival value that are suggestive of attachment include seeking proximity, separation distress and the secure base effect.

1.99   Weak opiates such as codeine are appropriate for use alongside monoamine oxidase inhibitors.

1.100 Spontaneous recovery is the reappearance of the conditioned stimulus without the conditioned response.

1.101 Hearing a running commentary is an example of a first-rank symptom that is pathognomonic of schizophrenia.

1.102 Dopamine is an excitatory neurotransmitter.

1.103 Hepatic phase I metabolism includes synthetic reactions.

1.104 Imprinting is seen in geese but not in humans.

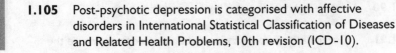

1.105 Post-psychotic depression is categorised with affective disorders in International Statistical Classification of Diseases and Related Health Problems, 10th revision (ICD-10).

1.106 Heroin use is associated with nasal septal defects.

1.107 Coprolalia can lead to hepatitis.

1.108 Suicidal thoughts and a desire to join the deceased are normal after bereavement.

1.109 When taking reversible inhibitors of monoamine oxidase A, it is safe to eat almost unlimited quantities of cheese.

1.110 Jung first defined the terms introversion and individuation.

1.111 Hepatic phase II metabolism includes synthetic reactions resulting in conjugation.

1.112 Command hallucinations must always be obeyed.

1.113 The balance theory of interpersonal attraction suggests that people with different beliefs reach a compromise and come to like one another.

1.114 High expressed emotion causes more frequent relapses in patients with schizophrenia and also those with depressive disorders.

1.115 Hypothetical reasoning is a feature of the preoperational stage.

1.116 All illusions are increased with inattention.

1.117 Drugs with first-order kinetics are eliminated in proportion to the amount of drug present.

1.118 Winnicott described factors that could lead to the development of a false self.

1.119 Twins experience a delay in language development compared with matched non-twins.

1.120 The International Statistical Classification of Diseases and Related Health Problems, 10th revision (ICD-10) classification system was developed by the American Psychiatric Association.

1.121 According to Piaget, schemata are unchanging beliefs that are central to our understanding of the world.

1.122 Cattell used oblique factor analysis.

1.123 Winnicott described holding environments which create a sense of safety and allow therapy to take place.

1.124 *Hypericum perforatum* has marked effects on cytochrome p450 enzymes.

1.125 A normal grief reaction progresses through a stage of initial shock or numbness, through sadness, to a resolution of symptoms.

1.126 Multiple spider naevi may indicate bulimia nervosa.

1.127 Object permanence develops during the sensorimotor stage of development, according to Piaget.

1.128 Drugs administered rectally are absorbed directly into the hepatic portal circulation.

1.129 Telegraphic speech includes use of nouns and adjectives at the expense of other parts of speech.

1.130 Humanism considers the scientific method to be the most appropriate means for studying humans and their behaviour.

1.131 Cognitive irrelevance describes two contrasting beliefs.

1.132 The minimax principle proposes essentially selfish reasons for maintaining friendships.

1.133 Piaget's formal operational stage of reasoning is achieved universally by 19 years.

EXTENDED MATCHING ITEMS

I.134 THEME: SYMPTOMS OF ILLICIT SUBSTANCE USE

A	Alcohol intoxication
B	Alcohol withdrawal
C	Amphetamine intoxication
D	Benzodiazepine intoxication
E	Caffeine withdrawal
F	Cannabis intoxication
G	Cocaine intoxication
H	Lysergic acid diethylamide (LSD) intoxication
I	Opiate intoxication
J	Opiate withdrawal

Which of the above is the most likely cause for each of the following:

1   A young man is brought to Accident and Emergency by his friend. He feels unwell, with malaise and rigors. He has been vomiting and has dilated pupils.

2   The ambulance crew brings an unconscious young woman into the hospital. She was found lying face down in a public toilet next to a syringe and is making very little respiratory effort.

3   A man calls the emergency services to ask for help. His friend has jumped from the roof of his block of flats after shouting to bystanders, telling them that everything was wonderful, that he could see the angels, and that he was going to fly to the moon.

1.135   THEME: MANAGEMENT OF ANTIPSYCHOTIC SIDE-EFFECTS

A	Change of antipsychotic to an oral typical antipsychotic
B	Change of antipsychotic to another atypical antipsychotic
C	Change of antipsychotic to clozapine
D	High-dose benzodiazepines
E	Intramuscular injection of an antimuscarinic drug
F	Long-acting injection of atypical antipsychotic
G	Methadone
H	Oral propranolol
I	Stop all medication
J	Typical antipsychotic depot injection

Choose the most appropriate management from the list above for each of the following scenarios:

1   A young man who develops facial discomfort and oropharyngeal spasm after his first dose of antipsychotic medication.

2   A middle-aged man who experiences progressive weight gain while taking an atypical antipsychotic and stops taking it.

3   A young woman with schizophrenia that has failed to respond to two appropriate courses of atypical antipsychotics, despite good compliance.

1.136 THEME: TRANSCULTURAL ASPECTS OF PSYCHIATRY

A   Amok
B   Brain fag syndrome
C   Dhat
D   Khat
E   Koro
F   Latah
G   Piblokto
H   Trance
I   Windigo

For each of the following, choose the most appropriate word from the list above:

1   Occurs in Malay men.
2   Involves the belief that the penis will retract into the abdomen.
3   Relates to concern about excessive masturbation.

1.137   THEME: DEPRESSIVE DISORDERS

A	Allport
B	Beck
C	Brown and Harris
D	Freud
E	Liddle
F	Pavlov
G	Schachter
H	Schildkraut
I	Vaughn and Leff

Choose the person from the list above who described each of the following in depression:

1   Cognitive errors
2   Vulnerability factors
3   High expressed emotion

1.138   THEME: PHYSICAL SIGNS

A	Battell's sign
B	Lanugo hair
C	Love's sign
D	Malar rash
E	Palmar erythema
F	Pyoderma gangrenosum
G	Russell's sign
H	Titubation
I	Turner's sign

Choose the most characteristic feature from the list above for each of the following:

1   Bulimia nervosa
2   Anorexia nervosa
3   Chronic alcohol abuse

1.139   THEME: FREUD'S THEORY OF DEVELOPMENT

A   Anal-expulsive stage
B   Anal-retentive stage
C   Depressive position
D   Electra complex
E   Genital phase
F   Latency period
G   Oral stage
H   Paranoid-schizoid position
I   Phallic-Oedipal stage

Choose the most appropriate stage from the list above for each of the following:

1   The stage during which an awareness of genitalia develops.
2   The stage immediately following the phallic-Oedipal stage.
3   The initial stage of development in Freudian theory.

1.140   THEME: KLEINIAN THEORY

A	Denial
B	Depressive position
C	Idealism
D	Introjection
E	Manic defence
F	Omnipotence
G	Paranoid-schizoid position
H	Projection
I	Projective identification

Choose the item from the list above most closely described by each of the following:

1   This develops during the first 6 months of life and is characterised by isolation and persecutory fears.

2   Objects are perceived as a whole and the world is appreciated as imperfect.

3   Bad objects undergo this process, which is a psychotic defence.

1.141 THEME: IDIOGRAPHIC PERSONALITY THEORY

A   Actualising tendency
B   Conditional positive regard
C   Conditions of worth
D   Ideal self
E   Incongruence
F   Perceived self
G   Phenomenal field
H   The trait approach
I   Unconditional positive regard

Identify the item from the list above most closely described by each of the following:

1   The difference between the ideal self and the perceived self.
2   This drives people to grow, develop and achieve their potential.
3   This is the most common view that others have of you as a person.

1.142 THEME: MOVEMENT DISORDERS

A	Akinesia
B	Athetosis
C	Chorea
D	Dystonia
E	Hyperkinesia
F	Myoclonus
G	Resting tremor
H	Spasmodic torticollis
I	Static tremor

Choose the movement disorder from the list above most associated with each of the following:

1   Depressive stupor
2   Creutzfeldt–Jakob disease
3   Generalised anxiety disorder

1.143   THEME: MORAL DEVELOPMENT

A	Anal-expulsive
B	Heteronomous stage (rigid moral development – 5–11 years)
C	Hypothetico-deductive reasoning
D	Initiative (4–5 years)
E	Morality of care (girls)
F	Morality of justice (boys)
G	Post-conventional morality (20+ years)
H	Precausal reasoning
I	Stage 3 – mutual role taking (10–12 years)

Identify the stage of moral development from the list above associated with each of the following:

1	Piaget
2	Selman
3	Kohlberg

PRACTICE PAPER 1

Answers

INDIVIDUAL STATEMENT QUESTIONS

1.1 **False** – It is a benzisoxamole. Dibenzazepines include clozapine and loxapine.
A–Z pp 34–8

1.2 **False** – It is more common in females.
A–Z pp 106–10

1.3 **True** – This is one of many approaches to the subject.
A–Z pp 217–18

1.4 **False** – It is rare, but not very rare. This seems like an academic distinction, but it has been tested in the exam several times.
A–Z pp 312–13

1.5 **False** – It is reduced.
A–Z pp 179–80

1.6 **False** – This describes the id.
A–Z p 308

1.7 **True** – This is an important first step.
A Guide to Psychiatric Examination p 53

1.8 **True** – The dose equivalents are listed in the British National Formulary and also in The A–Z of the MRCPsych.
A–Z pp 34–8

1.9 **True** – Although akathisia classically occurs early in treatment, it can occur very late and present in a way similar to tardive dyskinesia.
A–Z pp 140–2

1.10 **True** – Also toothache.
A–Z pp 312–13

1.11 **False** – It is the ability to differentiate between any object and the background.
A–Z p 146, Fear p 8

1.12 **True** – There is potential for a dangerous interaction.
Fear p162

1.13 **False** – It must be conscious to be recognised.
A–Z p 144

1.14 **False** – It has very little effect.
Fear p 149

1.15 **False** – They are particularly common in Lewy body dementia.
A–Z pp 97–8

1.16 **False** – Only fresh fish may be eaten.
A–Z pp 213–14

1.17 **False** – It is also known as *vorbeigehen*. *Vorbeireden* is also known as talking past the point.
A–Z p 332

1.18 **False** – They are determined by cognitive, affective and behavioural components. The behavioural component is also known as the conative component.
A–Z pp 50–1

1.19 **False** – The day residue and nocturnal stimuli, as well as unconscious wishes.
A–Z p 124

1.20 **False** – It is common and results from behaviour that contradicts one's internal beliefs.
A–Z p 119

1.21 **True** – The stage of identity vs confusion lasts

from 12 to 18 years.
A–Z pp 355–9

1.22   **True** – He considered it to lead to delinquency.
Fear p 51

1.23   **False** – Single women.
A–Z p 91

1.24   **False** – Freud used this expression.
A–Z p 124

1.25   **False** – This is a fundamental and important aspect of the psychiatric history.
A Guide to Psychiatric Examination pp 67–70

1.26   **False** – It involves factual knowledge.
A–Z p 207

1.27   **True** – This is widely reported.
A–Z p 157

1.28   **False** – They are involuntary.
A–Z pp 159–61

1.29   **True** – Failure of any component results in difficulties.
A–Z p 205, Fear p 13

1.30   **False** – It is the inability to understand the written word. The inability to recognise emotions is alexithymia.
Fear p 101

1.31   **False** – They are generally preferred, but there are some exceptions. Be wary of questions using the word 'always'.
A–Z pp 34–8

1.32   **False** – It is a primitive defence mechanism.
A–Z pp 92–3

1.33   **True** – Some also precipitates.
A–Z p 179

I.34   **True** – And should therefore be avoided with monoamine
oxidase inhibitors.
A–Z pp 213–14

I.35   **True** – They are highly suggestive of schizophrenia, but not
diagnostic.
A–Z p 293

I.36   **True** – It is also known as approximate answers.
A–Z p 332

I.37   **False** – Paraphrenia is not included.
A–Z pp 349–50

I.38   **False** – Foucault was an anti-psychiatrist, but Klein was a
prominent psychiatrist.
A–Z pp 148, 185

I.39   **True** – It is the process of storing groups of items rather than
individual items.
Fear p 13

I.40   **False** – Flumazenil is a GABA-A antagonist.
Fear p 153

I.41   **False** – The reverse is true.
A–Z p 75

I.42   **False** – The reverse is true.
A–Z p 102

I.43   **False** – It measures attitudes.
A–Z p 50

I.44   **True** – This is almost universally described.
A–Z pp 146–7, 201–2

I.45   **True** – It is a precursor for dihydroxyphenylalanine (DOPA)
and then dopamine.
A–Z pp 122–3

1.46 **False** – This is the concrete operational period. The preoperational stage lasts from approximately 2 to 7 years.
A–Z pp 254–5

1.47 **False** – There is no evidence to support this, although it is a common concern among trainees new to psychiatry.
A Guide to Psychiatric Examination pp 67–70

1.48 **False** – It has been observed in many species and plays a part in depression in humans.
A–Z pp 12–14, 192

1.49 **False** – It suggests that people who are elderly and belong to another minority are doubly disadvantaged.
A–Z pp 15–17

1.50 **True** – A purple tinge is reported.
A–Z pp 34–8

1.51 **False** – The coenestopathic state simply describes the constant awareness we have of the physical state of our own body.
A–Z p 76

1.52 **True** – This is the sensation of insects crawling over the skin.
A–Z p 148

1.53 **False** – Cream cheese and cottage cheese are safe to eat when taking monoamine oxidase inhibitors.
A–Z pp 213–14

1.54 **False** – It operates between thoughts.
A–Z p 104

1.55 **False** – It is a 5HT antagonist.
A–Z p 200

1.56 **True** – They often include headache and backache.
A–Z p 152

1.57 **False** – Many versions are available.
A–Z p 175

1.58   **False** – They were described by Kurt Schneider.
A–Z p 293

1.59   **False** – They result from the anti-α_1-adrenergic actions.
A–Z pp 34–8

1.60   **True** – This is also known as having a 'photographic memory'.
A–Z p 208

1.61   **False** – The pyrexia results from a central effect, but the dry
mouth results from peripheral antimuscarinic effects.
A–Z pp 34–8

1.62   **True**
A–Z p 202

1.63   **False** – The chairs should be at an angle to one another, to
reduce the level of anxiety the patient feels and enable both
the patient and examiner to take control over how much eye
contact is made.
A Guide to Psychiatric Examination pp 18–19

1.64   **False** – Change in one component causes change in the other
components and in the attitude as a whole.
A–Z p 50

1.65   **False** – They are usually poorly localised.
A–Z pp 159–60

1.66   **False** – An inaccuracy of an hour is typically allowed.
A–Z p 116

1.67   **True** – This is experienced as unpleasant.
A–Z p 39

1.68   **True** – There is a significant relationship.
A–Z p 144

1.69   **True** – It is almost entirely cleared by the kidney.
A–Z pp 195–7

1.70   **False** – The reverse is true.
A–Z pp 349–50

1.71   **False** – They are lipophilic and hydrophobic.
A–Z pp 31–4

1.72   **True** – This is hypersalivation.
A–Z pp 75–6

1.73   **True** – Also noradrenaline receptors.
A–Z pp 34–8

1.74   **True** – An example of a receptor antagonist with this effect is
mirtazapine.
Fear p 152

1.75   **True** – It is similar to adrenaline and noradrenaline in this
respect.
A–Z pp 122–3

1.76   **False** – Illusions follow a real perceptual experience, unlike
hallucinations.
A–Z p 176

1.77   **False** – It is a technique used to stop intrusive thoughts.
Thought sonalisation is synonymous with thought echo.
A–Z p 322

1.78   **False** – It is unconscious.
A–Z p 308

1.79   **False** – Long-term memory demands effort for retrieval,
whereas retrieval from short-term memory is almost effortless.
A–Z pp 208–9

1.80   **False** – This was Carl Schneider.
A–Z p 293

1.81   **False** – Disorientation in time occurs first, then in place and
finally in person.
A–Z p 116

1.82 **True** – The memory has usually been encoded and stored, but cannot be retrieved.
A–Z p 208

1.83 **False** – They are usually auditory.
A–Z p 160

1.84 **True** – Metoclopramide and antipsychotics have the same effect.
A–Z pp 122–3

1.85 **False** – They were described by Kurt Schneider.
A–Z p 293

1.86 **True** – Thorndike was influential before World War I and Skinner was active in the 1930s.
A–Z p 80

1.87 **False** – Affect is short-term and often directed to individuals or objects. Mood is longer term.
Fear pp 99–100

1.88 **False** – It causes positive feelings between people who are familiar with one another.
A–Z p 50

1.89 **True** – This is almost universally reported.
A–Z p 116

1.90 **False** – Antagonists block the receptor but have no other effect on the target cell. Inverse agonists have the opposite effects to agonists.
Fear p 152

1.91 **False** – All antipsychotics can cause it.
A–Z pp 75–6

1.92 **True** – They were therefore a unique insight into the unconscious mind.
A–Z p 124

1.93 **True** – They also tend to perform slightly less well at school. Fear p 358

1.94 **False** – They cause both. A–Z pp 34–8

1.95 **True**

1.96 **False** – This describes illusions. Hallucinations do not result from perceptual stimuli. A–Z p 176

1.97 **True** – Certain stimuli are more likely to induce a phobic response. A–Z pp 79–80

1.98 **True** – These were identified by Bowlby. A–Z pp 46–7

1.99 **False** – All opiates should be avoided. A–Z pp 213–14

1.100 **False** – It is the reappearance of the conditioned response without the unconditioned stimulus and follows a period of extinction, which is seen when the association between the conditioned and unconditioned stimuli is lost. A–Z p 79, Fear p 4

1.101 **False** – First-rank symptoms are highly suggestive of schizophrenia, but not pathognomonic. A–Z p 293

1.102 **False** – It is inhibitory. A–Z pp 122–3

1.103 **False** – It includes only non-synthetic reactions. A–Z pp 209–10

1.104 **True** – It is specific to certain species. A–Z p 177

1.105 **False** – It is categorised with schizophrenia, schizotypal and delusional disorders.
A–Z pp 349–50

1.106 **False** – These are a feature of cocaine use, when the cocaine is snorted.
A Guide to Psychiatric Examination pp 61–3

1.107 **False** – Coprolalia is the excessive use of obscene language. Coprophagia is the ingestion of faeces, which can cause hepatitis.
A–Z p 85

1.108 **False** – They indicate an abnormal grief reaction.
A–Z pp 155–6

1.109 **False** – There is still a risk of precipitating the cheese reaction with large amounts.
Fear p 163

1.110 **True** – Also extroversion.
A–Z pp 182–3

1.111 **True** – Creating a water soluble conjugate which can be excreted.
A–Z pp 209–10

1.112 **False** – They are usually ignored.
A–Z p 160

1.113 **False** – It suggests that only those with similar beliefs experience interpersonal attraction.
A–Z p 51

1.114 **True** – High expressed emotion was described by Vaughn and Leff.
A–Z pp 12–14

1.115 **False** – Hypothetical reasoning develops during the later formal operational stage.
A–Z pp 254–5

1.116 **False** – Pareidolic illusions increase with attention.
A–Z p 176

1.117 **True** – So the amount of drug eliminated in each half-life varies.
Fear p 145

1.118 **True** – Such as a pathological mother.
A–Z pp 333–4

1.119 **True** – There is a significant correlation.
A–Z p 144

1.120 **False** – It was developed by the World Health Organization.
A–Z p 175

1.121 **False** – They change in response to experience.
A–Z pp 253–5

1.122 **True** – Eysenck used orthogonal factor analysis.
A–Z pp 249–51

1.123 **True** – They are therapeutic settings.
A–Z pp 333–4

1.124 **True** – St John's Wort contains psychoactive substances
similar to those found in prescribed antidepressants.
Fear p 163

1.125 **True** – These are the three stages of grief reactions, as
described by Parkes.
A–Z pp 154–5

1.126 **False** – They are associated with alcoholism.
A Guide to Psychiatric Examination pp 61–3

1.127 **True** – Cognitive sequences also develop at this time.
Fear p 48

1.128 **False** – They are absorbed into the systemic circulation and
undergo little first-pass metabolism.
Fear p 147

1.129 **False** – Nouns and verbs.
Fear p 49

1.130 **False** – It considers cold science irrelevant to the study of complex, unique individuals.
A–Z p 167

1.131 **False** – It describes two beliefs that are unrelated.
A–Z p 119

1.132 **True** – It involves maximisation of reward and minimisation of cost relating to friendships.
A–Z pp 51–2

1.133 **False** – Although this level can be achieved by the age of 12 years, only a minority of people ever reach it.
A–Z pp 254–5

EXTENDED MATCHING ITEMS

1.134   THEME: SYMPTOMS OF ILLICIT SUBSTANCE USE

1   **J** – Opiate withdrawal.
2   **I** – Opiate intoxication.
3   **H** – LSD intoxication.
Fear pp 486–8, 490

1.135   THEME: MANAGEMENT OF ANTIPSYCHOTIC SIDE-EFFECTS

1   **E** – This is acute dystonia and should be treated by an intramuscular injection of an antimuscarinic drug. He may well be unable to swallow tablets
2   **B** – Change of antipsychotic to another atypical antipsychotic.
3   **C** – Change of antipsychotic to clozapine. She has treatment-resistant schizophrenia

1.136   THEME: TRANSCULTURAL ASPECTS OF PSYCHIATRY

1   **A** – Amok
2   **E** – Koro
3   **C** – Dhat
A–Z pp 361–3

1.137   THEME: DEPRESSIVE DISORDERS

1   **B** – Beck
2   **C** – Brown and Harris
3   **I** – Vaughn and Leff

1.138   THEME: PHYSICAL SIGNS

1   **G** – Russell's sign. This is callouses on the back of the fingers or hand from the repeated induction of vomiting with the hand
2   **B** – Lanugo hair
3   **E** – Palmar erythema. Due to hepatic involvement

1.139 THEME: FREUD'S THEORY OF DEVELOPMENT

1   I – Phallic-Oedipal stage
2   F – Latency period
3   G – Oral stage

1.140 THEME: KLEINIAN THEORY

1   G – Paranoid-schizoid position
2   B – Depressive position
3   I – Projective identification

A–Z pp 185–6

1.141 THEME: IDIOGRAPHIC PERSONALITY THEORY

1   E – Incongruence
2   A – Actualising tendency
3   B – Conditional positive regard

1.142 THEME: MOVEMENT DISORDERS

1   A – Akinesia
2   F – Myoclonus
3   I – Static tremor

Fear pp 96–7

1.143 THEME: MORAL DEVELOPMENT

1   B – Heteronomous stage (rigid moral development – 5–11
        years)
2   I – Stage 3 – mutual role taking (10–12 years)
3   G – Post-conventional morality (20+ years)

PRACTICE PAPER 2

Time allowed: 90 minutes

INDIVIDUAL STATEMENT QUESTIONS

2.1 Behaviour determines outcome in operant conditioning.

2.2 Illusions may occur secondary to hallucinations.

2.3 Tricyclic antidepressants can cause QT prolongation.

2.4 Alzheimer's disease is characterised by relative preservation of memory.

2.5 The risk of a pathological grief reaction is increased if the bereaved is grieving for another person at the time of the death.

2.6 A history of several hospital admissions in childhood is a risk factor for conduct disorder later in childhood.

2.7 A period of rapid vocabulary gain occurs at about 18 months.

2.8 Anhedonia is a state entirely devoid of affect.

2.9 Dopamine concentrations correlate positively with prolactin concentrations.

2.10 Photographic memory is more common in children than adults.

2.11 Masters and Johnson described three stages of sexual response – excitement, plateau and orgasm.

2.12 Normal syntactic structure of speech is more suggestive of schizophrenia than of mania.

2.13 Harlow worked mainly with baboons, studying aggressive drives and mechanisms of social dominance.

2.14 Attribution theory predicts a bias towards internal or dispositional attribution.

2.15 Metabolism of drugs can start in the stomach cavity.

2.16 Disturbance of gait is common in Alzheimer's disease.

2.17 Short-term visual memory is located in the right hemisphere.

2.18 Stigma develops during Freud's anal stage.

2.19 Repression is an effective means of totally eradicating painful memories, so that they have no further influence on an individual.

2.20 Transitional objects were first described by Freud.

2.21 Fear of negative evaluation increases at the time of puberty.

2.22 Unipolar depression involves the individual in a state reminiscent of the depressive position.

2.23 Illusions are a feature of temporal lobe epilepsy.

2.24 Argyll and Bute proposed rules of friendship.

2.25 Eidetic imagery requires voluntary recall to appear.

2.26 Jung described archetypes including the Great Mother, the Wise Old Man and the Original Tree.

2.27 De Clerambault's syndrome is usually associated with persistent delusional disorders.

2.28 The tuberoinfundibular system is characterised by a predominance of γ-amino butyric acid activated (GABAergic) neurotransmission.

2.29 5-Hydroxytryptamine 2A ($5HT_{2A}$) receptors are mainly presynaptic.

2.30   Loading doses of a drug must be used if the plasma steady state is ever to be achieved.

2.31   Patient-rated scales include the Hospital Anxiety and Depression Scale and the Leyton Obsessive Inventory.

2.32   Ribot's law of memory regression states that we can remember childhood events more clearly during times of physical illness.

2.33   Delusional perception is a second-rank symptom of schizophrenia.

2.34   It is not possible to test both long- and short-term memory during the same interview.

2.35   Winnicott described the good-enough mother.

2.36   Late insomnia is characteristic of generalised anxiety disorder.

2.37   Obsessive-compulsive disorder has equal sex incidence.

2.38   Clouding of consciousness may indicate a serious medical problem.

2.39   Auditory agnosia is seen in people with no hearing.

2.40   Morbid jealousy can be ignored, as it is self-limiting and rarely problematic.

2.41   Alcoholic hallucinosis usually involves seeing little people and animals.

2.42   The law of effect states that behaviours that result in positive experiences are more likely to be repeated.

2.43   Metabolised drug products with a molecular mass of 300 or more are usually excreted by the kidney.

2.44   Dopamine receptor antagonists have an emetic action.

2.45   Hallucinations only occur in the presence of a real external stimulus.

2.46   Excessive use of cocaine can lead to the development of morbid jealousy.

2.47   The rapid action of a drug after intravenous administration is always an advantage.

2.48   Female friendships are based on mutual understanding and emotional support.

2.49   Dopamine D2, D3 and D4 receptors are similar.

2.50   Cognition includes memory, language, thought and selective attention.

2.51   General medical conditions are classified on axis V in The Diagnostic and Statistical Manual of Mental Disorders-IV (DSM-IV).

2.52   Extracampine hallucinations can be heard by others.

2.53   Dopamine is a precursor of noradrenaline.

2.54   Morbid jealousy has been explained in terms of repressed homosexuality.

2.55   The Hawthorne effect describes the tendency of patients to get better, regardless of their treatment.

2.56   The James–Lange theory of emotion stresses the cognitive aspects of emotion.

2.57   People with visual agnosia can recognise objects by touch but not by sight.

2.58   Hallucinations are easily distinguishable from real perceptions.

2.59   Dissocial personality disorder typically involves impulsive actions within the context of a long-term, loving relationship, which increases the guilt felt subsequently.

2.60 Hearing one's own thoughts repeated aloud is known as *gedankenlautwerden*.

2.61 Capgras' syndrome, also known as the illusion of doubles, is actually a delusional perception.

2.62 Autoscopy involves seeing one's own body.

2.63 Post-traumatic amnesia correlates with later psychiatric disability after head injury.

2.64 Florid delusions are a feature of some hypothyroid states.

2.65 Tricyclic antidepressants are metabolised more slowly with age.

2.66 Magnification is helpful in management of depressive states.

2.67 McClelland described the need for achievement.

2.68 The second stage of development according to Piaget's theory starts at the age of 7 years.

2.69 Post-traumatic stress disorder is common after childbirth.

2.70 Capgras' syndrome often involves the spouse.

2.71 The need for intimacy is a motivation towards friendship.

2.72 Circumstantiality is more suggestive of schizophrenia than of mania.

2.73 Classical conditioning causes association between a voluntary response and a stimulus not normally associated with it.

2.74 An emotional response is composed of subjective awareness, physiological changes and cognitive-behavioural elements.

2.75 Imagery is under voluntary control.

2.76 Metabolism occurs in the skin to a limited extent.

2.77 Personal construct theory is well suited for the investigation of unconscious traits.

2.78 Winnicott felt that it was normal for a mother to have feelings of hatred for her child from the start of their relationship.

2.79 The predominant defence mechanism in the development of hysterical symptoms is denial.

2.80 Lithium, as used therapeutically, is highly lipid soluble.

2.81 Hallucinations of little people are known as reflex hallucinations.

2.82 Persistent delusional disorder typically features bizarre delusions.

2.83 Ganser's syndrome was originally described in soldiers.

2.84 Thought blocking is synonymous with thought withdrawal.

2.85 Delusions in Lewy body dementia are often systematised.

2.86 Perceptual abilities of animals can be investigated using conditioned discrimination.

2.87 Tricyclics do not bind to plasma proteins.

2.88 Couvade syndrome is associated with ambivalence about fatherhood.

2.89 Most lithium is metabolised by the liver.

2.90 D1 and D4 receptors are structurally similar.

2.91 Lithium has a high therapeutic index which necessitates plasma monitoring.

2.92 Obsessive-compulsive disorder is most common in lower social classes.

2.93 Illusions include mirage, macropsia and *jamais vu*.

2.94 Extrapyramidal side-effects cause a parkinsonian picture, but without the classical pill-rolling tremor.

2.95 Schachter described the cognitive labelling theory of emotion.

2.96 The friends of preschool children are selected by adults.

2.97 Democratic leadership is the most effective type when highly creative tasks need to be completed.

2.98 Males have more verbally oriented friendships than females.

2.99 It has been suggested that children learn aggressive behaviour from the television as a result of sensitisation to violence.

2.100 Hallucinations can feature in persistent delusional disorder.

2.101 It is advisable to be cautious when asking patients about suicide, and not to indicate which of the methods they have considered are likely to be successful.

2.102 Haptic hallucinations are located deep within the body, usually within the abdomen.

2.103 Prejudice is enacted discrimination.

2.104 Hallucinations are perceptions without an object.

2.105 γ-Amino butyric acid (GABA) is pro-convulsant.

2.106 Autocratic leadership is more effective than democratic leadership in most situations.

2.107 Depersonalisation is unpleasant.

2.108 Chronic antagonists typically cause downregulation of receptors.

2.109 The three types of adverse drug reaction include intolerance, allergic reactions and drug interactions.

2.110   The oral contraceptive pill reduces the action of tricyclic antidepressants.

2.111   All recognised disorders are categorised in the International Statistical Classification of Diseases and Related Health Problems, 10th revision (ICD-10).

2.112   Younger children are significantly less intellectually developed compared with their oldest sibling at the same age.

2.113   The strange situation experiment was classically conducted on a 3-year-old child.

2.114   Bandura described direct tuition and classical conditioning as the two forms of social learning.

2.115   Capgras' syndrome is more common in men than women.

2.116   Attachment is extinguished by the time of adulthood.

2.117   Leaders typically feel more need for dominance than others.

2.118   Lewy body dementia features bradykinesia, tremor and rigidity.

2.119   Feeling unrefreshed after sleep is reported by patients with generalised anxiety disorder.

2.120   Much of the cardiotoxicity of tricyclic antidepressants results from their effects on serotonin activity.

2.121   Morbid jealousy is also known as Capgras' syndrome.

2.122   Reduction of γ-amino butyric acid (GABA) concentrations leads to a reduction of anxiety levels.

2.123   The anxious/avoidant child does not appear distressed at the mother's departure during the strange situation experiment and may play with the stranger.

2.124 The Diagnostic and Statistical Manual of Mental Disorders-IV (DSM-IV) has three axes.

2.125 Visual hallucinations are often a feature of Lewy body dementia.

2.126 Depersonalisation is pathognomonic of mental illness.

2.127 In Pavlov's classic experiment with dogs, the bell represented the unconditioned stimulus and the food represented the conditioned stimulus.

2.128 Reciprocal inhibition is used to treat anxiety.

2.129 Over 90% of infants are securely attached at 1 year.

2.130 The development of anxiety after exposure to environmental stimuli is explained by operant conditioning.

2.131 Over-valued ideas can be eliminated by reasoned argument.

2.132 A securely attached child is distressed at its mother's departure during the strange situation experiment but seeks proximity when she returns, despite a show of anger.

2.133 Fathers typically sit further from their children than mothers.

EXTENDED MATCHING ITEMS

2.134   THEME: FALSE PERCEPTIONS

A   Affect illusion
B   Completion illusion
C   Ecmnesiac hallucinations
D   Extracampine hallucinations
E   Functional hallucinations
F   Haptic hallucinations
G   Imagery
H   Kinaesthetic hallucinations
I   Pareidolic illusion
J   Reflex hallucinations

Choose the descriptive term from the above list that is most appropriate for the following:

1   Hearing whispering voices whenever the wind can be heard blowing through the trees.
2   The limbs are felt to be twisting and deformed.
3   The sensation that the skin is being pricked with pins, believed to be the result of punishment by invisible demons.

2.135   THEME: RECEPTOR ANTAGONISM

A   α-Adrenoceptors
B   β$_1$-Adrenoceptors
C   γ-Amino butyric acid (GABA)-A
D   γ-Amino butyric acid (GABA)-B
E   D1 receptors
F   D2 receptors
G   5-Hydroxytryptamine (5HT)$_1$ receptors
H   Muscarinic acetylcholinergic receptors
I   Nicotinic acetylcholinergic receptors

Choose the receptor from the list above which is the site of antagonism of each of the following:

1   Propranolol
2   Atropine
3   Flumazenil

2.136   THEME: CLINICAL FEATURES OF ANXIETY DISORDERS

A	Acute stress reaction
B	Adjustment disorder
C	Agoraphobia
D	Diogenes' syndrome
E	Generalised anxiety disorder
F	Moderate depressive episode
G	Panic disorder
H	Post-traumatic stress disorder
I	Social phobia

Choose the disorder from the list above most closely associated with each of the following:

1   Discrete episodes of severe anxiety accompanied by fear of imminent death.
2   Anticipatory anxiety and a reluctance to leave home.
3   A 3-day history of anxiety and depression after surviving a plane crash.

2.137   THEME: DISORDER OF THOUGHT

A	Depressive disorder
B	Epilepsy
C	Generalised anxiety disorder
D	Mania
E	Obsessive-compulsive disorder
F	Persistent delusional disorder
G	Post-traumatic stress disorder
H	Schizophrenia
I	Schizotypal disorder

Choose the disorder from the list above most associated with each of the following:

1   Clanging, distractibility and circumstantiality.
2   Substitution, derailment, drivelling and fusion.
3   Poverty of speech.

2.138 THEME: NOMOTHETIC PERSONALITY THEORY

A	Factor analytic randomisation
B	First order factors
C	L data
D	Oblique factor analysis
E	Orthogonal factor analysis
F	Q data
G	State approaches
H	T data
I	5 Universal factors

Identify the item from the list above as described below:

1   The technique used by Eysenck to identify a small number of independent factors.

2   The personality descriptions derived by use of questionnaires based on primary traits.

3   The most important aspects of personality, as described by Costa and McCrea.

2.139   THEME: MOVEMENT DISORDER

A   Akathisia
B   Akinesia
C   Athetosis
D   Essential tremor
E   Flapping tremor
F   Hyperkinesia
G   Resting tremor
H   Static tremor
I   Tic

Choose the movement disorder from the list above most commonly resulting from treatment with each of the following:

1   Lithium
2   Selective serotonin reuptake inhibitors
3   Antipsychotics

2.140   THEME: THEORISTS

A	Adler
B	Bleuler
C	Freud
D	Janov
E	Klein
F	Reich
G	Rogers
H	Schneider
I	Winnicott

Identify the theorist from the list above who described:

1   Primal therapy
2   The will to power
3   The organ energy accumulator

2.141 THEME: PERSONALITY THEORISTS

A	Allport
B	Bandura
C	Cattell
D	Eysenck
E	Freud
F	Jung
G	Klein
H	Rogers
I	Skinner

Identify the individual from the list above who is most associated with the following:

1 Humanistic theory
2 Operant conditioning
3 Modelling

2.142   THEME: BEREAVEMENT

A	Depression
B	Encopresis
C	Functional enuresis
D	Hallucinations
E	Late insomnia
F	Mania
G	Prolonged sadness
H	Thought disorder
I	Weight loss of more than 15% of total body weight

Identify the item from the list above which:

1   Was described by Parkes as one of the five stages of bereavement.
2   Is a feature of bereavement in young children.
3   Is part of the initial bereavement reaction when a child's parent dies.

2.143 THEME: AMNESIA

A	Amnesia of Korsakoff's syndrome
B	Catathymic amnesia
C	Diencephalic amnesia
D	Dysmnesic syndrome
E	Hippocampal amnesia
F	Post-hypnotic amnesia
G	Post-traumatic amnesia
H	Psychogenic amnesia
I	Retrograde amnesia
J	Transient global amnesia

Choose the correct type of amnesia from the list above for each of the following:

1   Often related to head injury, this type of amnesia is a relatively good predictor of final clinical outcome.
2   Associated with criminal behaviour and crises relating to relationships, this type of amnesia causes global amnesia for specific events.
3   This describes the type of amnesia relating to painful, repressed memories.

PRACTICE PAPER 2

Answers

INDIVIDUAL STATEMENT QUESTIONS

2.1   **True** – This contrasts with classical conditioning, where
stimuli determine outcome.
A–Z p 80

2.2   **True** – This results in delusional illusions.
A–Z p 176

2.3   **True** – And a risk of serious arrhythmias.
A–Z pp 31–4

2.4   **False** – There is marked memory disturbance from the onset.
A–Z pp 106–10

2.5   **True**
A–Z pp 155–6

2.6   **True** – Although the reasons for this are unclear.
Fear p 358

2.7   **True** – This is helped by naming games.
A–Z pp 190–1

2.8   **False** – It is unpleasant by definition and therefore has an
affective component.
A–Z p 26

2.9   **False** – There is a negative correlation. Dopamine released in
the hypothalamic–hypophyseal pathway reduces prolactin
secretion. Antipsychotics antagonise the action of dopamine
here and cause hyperprolactinaemia.
A–Z pp 122–3

2.10   **True** – Also known as eidetic imagery.
A–Z p 208

2.11   **False** – There is a fourth – resolution.
A–Z p 298

2.12   **False** – It is more suggestive of mania.
A–Z p 202

2.13   **False** – The work was done with infant chimpanzees, on attachment.
A–Z pp 162–3

2.14   **True** – This means that actions are attributed to people and their behaviour rather than to external factors beyond our control; it is known as the primary or fundamental attribution error.
A–Z p 52

2.15   **True** – Both stomach enzymes and stomach flora are involved.
Fear p 149

2.16   **True** – This is a common feature.
A–Z pp 106–10

2.17   **True** – And short-term verbal memory in the left hemisphere.
A–Z p 209

2.18   **False** – During the latent stage.
A–Z p 306

2.19   **False** – Although repressed memories cannot be recalled, they may manifest in other ways, such as neuroses.
A–Z pp 92–3

2.20   **False** – They were described by Winnicott.
A–Z p 227

2.21   **True** – This is also associated with social phobia.
A–Z p 145

2.22   **True** – Although the original depressive position is not pathological and unipolar depression is.
A–Z p 8–12

2.23   **True** – And of normal mental states.
A–Z p 176

2.24   **False** – It was Argyll and Henderson.
A–Z pp 149–50

2.25   **True** – It is also known as 'photographic memory'.
A–Z p 208

2.26   **False** – Not the Original Tree.
A–Z pp 182–3

2.27   **False** – It is usually associated with paranoid schizophrenia.
A–Z p 91

2.28   **False** – It is a dopamine system.
A–Z pp 122–3

2.29   **False** – They are mainly postsynaptic.
Fear p 156

2.30   **False** – They are not necessary, but do speed the process up.
Fear p 146

2.31   **False** – The Leyton Obsessive Inventory is clinician-rated.
Fear p 276

2.32   **False** – It states that memory for recent events is lost more
quickly in dementing illnesses.
Fear p 109

2.33   **False** – It is a first-rank symptom.
A–Z p 293

2.34   **False** – It is very helpful to test both of these routinely.
A Guide to Psychiatric Examination pp 56–7

2.35   **True** – This described a mother who was not over-involved.
A–Z pp 333–4

2.36   **False** – It is characteristic of a depressive disorder. Sleep
disorder in generalised anxiety disorder consists of initial
insomnia and waking during the night.
A–Z pp 114–15

2.37   **True** – This is true overall, but some presentations of the
disorder are more common in men or in women.
A–Z pp 230–1

2.38   **True** – It is important that relevant physical investigations are
carried out.
A–Z p 83

2.39   **False** – Agnosia occurs despite intact sensory pathways.
A–Z p 18

2.40   **False** – It is very important, as it is strongly associated with
serious violence.
A–Z p 181

2.41   **False** – This describes Lilliputian hallucinations which occur in
delirium tremens (and therefore clouded consciousness).
Alcoholic hallucinosis usually involves threatening voices.
A–Z p 162

2.42   **True** – Behaviours resulting in negative experiences are less
likely to be repeated.
Fear p 5

2.43   **False** – This is the threshold for excretion in bile.
A–Z pp 209–10

2.44   **False** – They are antiemetic and include metoclopramide and
antipsychotics.
A–Z pp 122–3

2.45   **False** – This describes illusions. Hallucinations occur without
perceptual stimuli.
A–Z pp 159–60

2.46   **True** – Although this is uncommon.
A–Z p 181

2.47   **False** – Some drugs, such as antipsychotic depot injections, are administered via the intramuscular route to prolong their duration of action.
A–Z pp 179–80

2.48   **True** – Male friendships are based on shared activities.
A–Z pp 149–50

2.49   **True** – They form a subgroup within the wider family of dopamine receptors.
A–Z pp 122–3

2.50   **True** – Also perception.
A–Z p 76

2.51   **False** – They are classified on axis III. Axis V is for global assessment of function.
A–Z p 126

2.52   **False** – They are located outside the sensory field.
A–Z p 160

2.53   **True** – The process of dopamine production and breakdown is a common topic for questions in the exam.
A–Z pp 122–3

2.54   **True** – Although the truth of this is unclear.
A–Z p 181

2.55   **False** – It is the effect seen when the presence of an interviewer alters responses.
A–Z p 204

2.56   **False** – It emphasises the physical aspects.
A–Z p 181

2.57   **True** – Despite adequate eyesight.
A–Z p 18

2.58   **False** – They are subjectively identical to real percepts.
A–Z pp 159–60

2.59   **False** – Long-term, loving relationships are rarely achieved by people with dissocial personality disorder. Guilt is also rare.
A–Z pp 116–17

2.60   **True** – It is a first-rank symptom of schizophrenia.
A–Z p 160

2.61   **True** – Involving the belief that someone has been replaced by an impostor.
A–Z p 70

2.62   **True** – Seeing it from outside, but receiving sensory input (apart from visual input) as if one were still in the body that can be seen.
Fear p 99

2.63   **True** – There is a relatively good correlation.
A–Z p 24

2.64   **True** – In cases where an organic psychosis results.
A–Z p 173

2.65   **True** – So the dose may need to be reduced in the elderly.
A–Z pp 31–4

2.66   **False** – It refers to the cognitive error which magnifies one's own problems and contributes to depression.
A–Z p 201

2.67   **True** – And stressed aggressive drives.
A–Z p 204

2.68   **False** – It is the preoperational stage and it starts at the age of 2 years.
A–Z p 359

2.69   **False** – This is not the case.
A–Z pp 260–3

2.70   **True** – This is characteristic.
A–Z p 70

2.71   **True** – Together with the need for affiliation.
A–Z pp 149–50

2.72   **False** – It is more suggestive of mania.
A–Z p 202

2.73   **False** – The response must be an involuntary response or a
reflex, for example salivation.
A–Z p 79

2.74   **True** – But it is disputed by the James–Lange theory and the
Cannon–Bard theory.
A–Z pp 132–3

2.75   **True** – It is not perceived as real.
A–Z p 176

2.76   **True** – Other unusual sites include the lungs and placenta.
A–Z pp 209–10

2.77   **False** – It can only investigate conscious aspects of the
personality.
A–Z pp 247–9

2.78   **True** – He called this 'countertransference hate'.
A–Z pp 333–4

2.79   **True** – But the repressed distress is experienced in another
form.
A–Z p 173

2.80   **False** – It is highly water soluble.
A–Z p 195–7

2.81   **False** – They are Lilliputian hallucinations.
A–Z p 160

2.82 **False** – The delusions are usually not bizarre.
A–Z pp 113–14

2.83 **False** – It was originally described in prisoners.
A–Z p 152

2.84 **False** – They are different.
A–Z p 322

2.85 **True** – They are also difficult to treat because of sensitivity to antipsychotics.
A–Z pp 97–8

2.86 **True** – Bees can be conditioned to prefer red flowers over blue flowers. This demonstrates that they can discriminate between red and blue.
A–Z p 80

2.87 **False** – They are strongly bound to plasma proteins.
A–Z pp 31–4

2.88 **True** – Although there is no established relationship with poor parenting.
A–Z pp 312–13

2.89 **False** – It is excreted by the kidney.
A–Z pp 195–7

2.90 **False** – D1 and D5 receptors are similar.
A–Z pp 122–3

2.91 **False** – It has a low therapeutic index.
Fear p 146, A–Z pp 195-7

2.92 **False** – It is more common in higher social classes.
A–Z p 230–1

2.93 **True** – Also diplopia and *déjà vu*.
A–Z p 176

2.94   **False** – The pill-rolling tremor is seen.
A–Z pp 140–2

2.95   **True** – This is a relatively sophisticated theory.
A–Z pp 132–3

2.96   **True** – The child has little influence.
A–Z p 242

2.97   **False** – This is the only situation in which *laissez-faire*
leadership is useful.
A–Z p 192

2.98   **False** – The reverse is true.
A–Z pp 149–50

2.99   **False** – Desensitisation to violence may occur.
A–Z p 17

2.100   **True** – But they only fit within the definition if they relate to
the delusion.
A–Z pp 113–14

2.101   **True** – Many patients think that a small overdose (twice their
usual dose of antipsychotic, for example) will be immediately
fatal. It may not be helpful to give information to the contrary,
which may be taken by the patient as advice on how to harm
themselves most effectively.
A Guide to Psychiatric Examination pp 67–70

2.102   **False** – This describes visceral hallucinations. Haptic
hallucinations are superficial.
A–Z p 161

2.103   **False** – Discrimination is the act that follows the internal
beliefs called prejudice.
A–Z pp 105–6

2.104   **True** – This was Esquirol's definition.
A–Z pp 159–60

2.105 **False** – It is anticonvulsant.
A–Z p 151

2.106 **False** – It is only better in situations of urgency.
A–Z p 192

2.107 **True** – By definition, it is markedly unpleasant.
A–Z pp 101–2

2.108 **False** – They often cause upregulation of receptors, as seen with dopamine receptors after long-term antipsychotic use.
Fear p 152

2.109 **False** – The fourth type is idiosyncratic reactions.
A–Z pp 274–5

2.110 **True** – So the dose may need to be increased.
A–Z pp 31–4

2.111 **False** – Some important disorders such as dementia with Lewy bodies are not included.
A–Z pp 349–50

2.112 **True** – There is a slight but significant association between being the eldest sibling and having a higher intelligence quotient (IQ).
A–Z p 144

2.113 **False** – The child was 1 year old.
A–Z pp 306–8

2.114 **False** – Direct tuition and observational learning. Classical conditioning is not a form of social learning.
Fear p 50

2.115 **False** – It is more common in women.
A–Z p 70

2.116 **False** – It is lifelong and increases at times of illness or distress.
A–Z p 47

2.117 **True** – They are also more talkative than others.
A–Z p 192

2.118 **True** – Other parkinsonian features are also seen.
A–Z pp 97–8

2.119 **True** – This a relatively common.
A–Z pp 114–15

2.120 **True** – Their antiserotoninergic activity causes membrane stabilisation and therefore cardiac conduction abnormalities.
A–Z pp 31–4

2.121 **False** – It is also known as Othello syndrome. Capgras' syndrome is known as the illusion of doubles.
A–Z pp 181–2

2.122 **False** – The reverse is true.
A–Z p 151

2.123 **True** – This correlates with poor social function in later life.
A–Z pp 306–8

2.124 **False** – It has five axes.
A–Z p 126

2.125 **True** – They are usually elaborate and recurrent.
A–Z pp 97–8

2.126 **False** – It is an uncommon feature of normal experience.
A–Z pp 101–2

2.127 **False** – The bell was the conditioned stimulus and the food the unconditioned stimulus.
Fear pp 3–4

2.128 **True** – It involves relaxing to prevent anxiety, followed by exposure to anxiogenic stimuli.
A–Z p 178

2.129   **False** – The proportion is approximately 60%.
         Fear pp 508–10

2.130   **True** – This explains the development of many phobic
         disorders.
         A–Z pp 80–2

2.131   **True** – Unlike delusions.
         A–Z pp 175–6

2.132   **True** – The child will be reluctant to interact with the
         stranger.
         A–Z p 307

2.133   **True** – They also talk in more adult language and play more
         vigorously.
         A–Z p 144

EXTENDED MATCHING ITEMS

2.134 THEME: FALSE PERCEPTIONS

1 **E** – Functional hallucinations occur in association with an unrelated stimulus in the same modality
2 **H** – Kinaesthetic hallucinations are characteristic of schizophrenia
3 **F** – Haptic hallucinations are superficial and usually have a delusional element

A–Z pp 159–61

2.135 THEME: RECEPTOR ANTAGONISM

1 **B** – β_1-Adrenoceptors
2 **H** – Muscarinic acetylcholinergic receptors
3 **C** – γ-Amino butyric acid (GABA)-A

2.136 THEME: CLINICAL FEATURES OF ANXIETY DISORDERS

1 **G** – Panic disorder
2 **C** – Agoraphobia
3 **A** – Acute stress reaction

2.137 THEME: DISORDER OF THOUGHT

1 **D** – Mania
2 **H** – Schizophrenia. Along with omission, all these were described by Carl Schneider
3 **A** – Depressive disorder

2.138 THEME: NOMOTHETIC PERSONALITY THEORY

1 **E** – Orthogonal factor analysis
2 **F** – Q data
3 **I** – 5 Universal factors

A–Z pp 249–51

PAPER 2
ANSWERS

2.139 THEME: MOVEMENT DISORDER

1   H – Static tremor
2   B – Akinesia
3   A – Akathisia
Fear pp 96–7

2.140 THEME: THEORISTS

1   **D** – Janov
2   **A** – Adler
3   **F** – Reich

2.141 THEME: PERSONALITY THEORISTS

1   **H** – Rogers
2   **I** – Skinner
3   **B** – Bandura

2.142 THEME: BEREAVEMENT

1   **A** – Depression. The five are alarm, numbness, pining, depression and recovery/reorganisation
2   **C** – Functional enuresis. Also temper tantrums
3   **G** – Prolonged sadness

2.143 THEME: AMNESIA

1   **F** – Post-hypnotic amnesia. This is amnesia for the period just after the head injury
2   **H** – Psychogenic amnesia
3   **B** – Catathymic amnesia
A–Z pp 23–4

PRACTICE PAPER 3

Time allowed: 90 minutes

INDIVIDUAL STATEMENT QUESTIONS

3.1   Depersonalisation is a cognitive error contributing to depression.

3.2   Adler described overcompensation as trying too hard to overcome inferiority.

3.3   Anticipatory anxiety is a feature of phobias.

3.4   Completion illusions increase during inattention and result in partial shapes being perceived as whole.

3.5   Baclofen acts as an antagonist at γ-amino butyric acid (GABA)-A receptors.

3.6   The amyloid precursor protein gene is present on chromosome 18.

3.7   Perseveration is pathognomonic of functional psychiatric disorder.

3.8   Kelly's personal construct theory considers individuals to be engaged in experiments in order to reach conclusions about their world.

3.9   SANS assessed levels of sadness and neurosis.

3.10   Highly lipid soluble drugs tend to be absorbed more slowly after intramuscular administration than less lipid soluble drugs.

3.11   Lithium, when prepared for clinical use, is highly lipid soluble.

3.12   The placebo effect is most pronounced with very large or very small tablets.

3.13   Depersonalisation is usually associated with derealisation.

3.14 Mannerisms are goal-directed.

3.15 The James–Lange theory of emotion suggests that every emotion has a distinct physiological state associated with it.

3.16 Closure is a concept central to Gestalt principles of perception.

3.17 Dopamine is found in relative abundance in the cerebellum.

3.18 A loss of sense of purpose or meaning in life, accompanied by a history of behaviour characteristic of a recently deceased relative indicate a pathological grief reaction.

3.19 The motivation for negativism is usually clear.

3.20 Learned helplessness is explained by operant conditioning.

3.21 Half-lives are fixed in relation to drugs with zero-order kinetics.

3.22 Affect illusions are often mood congruent.

3.23 γ-Amino butyric acid (GABA) is a widespread excitatory neurotransmitter.

3.24 D3 receptors are commonly found in the cerebellum.

3.25 Alzheimer's disease accounts for up to 25% of all cases of dementia.

3.26 D2 and D5 receptors are similar.

3.27 Drugs with a low relative molecular mass are absorbed slowly after intramuscular administration.

3.28 The ego-ideal represents the more positive aspect of the id.

3.29 Brief hallucinations and social withdrawal indicate a pathological grief reaction.

3.30 Perceptual constancy ensures that we perceive objects as unchanging and constant despite changes in their appearance such as the object getting larger.

3.31 Schaffer described the interactions between an infant and a caregiver as being characterised by mutual animosity.

3.32 Finger agnosia is a feature of Gerstmann's syndrome.

3.33 Depersonalisation is always associated with derealisation.

3.34 Illusions are indicative of mental disorder.

3.35 Perseveration is the inappropriate repetition of speech.

3.36 A comprehensive and universally accepted theory has been advanced to explain altruistic behaviour.

3.37 Monozygous twin concordance for schizophrenia is 45%.

3.38 Uncomfortable postures are only ever maintained for short periods of time during states of waxy flexibility.

3.39 Vascular dementia often presents suddenly and may be associated with falls.

3.40 Factor analysis was central to idiographic personality theories.

3.41 Escape conditioning is a type of negative reinforcement.

3.42 Logorrhoea is a feature of catatonic states seen in schizophrenia.

3.43 Perseveration typically occurs in clear consciousness.

3.44 St John's Wort is safe to take alongside conventional antidepressants.

3.45 Logoclonia only occurs in schizophrenia.

3.46 Anticoagulant use is a relative contraindication to oral drug administration.

3.47 Allport and Rogers were both idiographic personality theorists.

3.48 Palilalia is a form of perseveration.

3.49 Nomothetic approaches to personality consider individuals to be unique.

3.50 Gender identity disorder features cross-dressing in childhood.

3.51 The extent of dopaminergic receptor binding of an antipsychotic correlates with its efficacy.

3.52 DSM stands for the Diagnostic and Statutory Manual of Mental Disorders.

3.53 Post-traumatic amnesia relates to the time between the injury and the last recalled memory before the injury.

3.54 Depersonalisation occurs in panic attacks and temporal lobe epilepsy, but never in normal mental states.

3.55 Physical examination of psychiatric patients is most appropriately conducted by general physicians or general practitioners as they have more expertise in this area than psychiatrists.

3.56 Ambiguous figures are difficult to differentiate from the background.

3.57 The reliability of psychiatric diagnosis is improved by the use of operational criteria.

3.58 Palilalia is a feature of catatonia.

3.59 Groupthink describes the tendency of groups to equivocate and fail to reach a decision due to a wish to incorporate the beliefs of all their members.

3.60   Agnosia is the inability to interpret sensory stimuli due to disruption to sensory pathways.

3.61   Operant conditioning is the process by which an involuntary behaviour is followed by a positive or negative event, which leads to a subsequent increase or reduction in the behaviour.

3.62   Depersonalisation is an example of a delusion.

3.63   Iconic memory has a longer duration than echoic memory.

3.64   Lithium has sedative effects.

3.65   Jung was the first to describe cognitive dissonance.

3.66   Over-valued ideas are fixed, false beliefs that persist despite evidence to the contrary, and which are not appropriate to the patient's educational, cultural or religious background.

3.67   Idiographic approaches to personality are person-centred.

3.68   Logical connections between thoughts are lost in circumstantial thinking.

3.69   Somatic expression of symptoms, as in hysteria and conversion disorders, is more common in people from lower social classes and those with low educational achievements.

3.70   Stranger anxiety develops at 2 months.

3.71   Patient-rated scales are more accurate.

3.72   Delayed conditioning involves an optimal delay of 2.5 s between presentation of the conditioned and unconditioned stimuli.

3.73   Prolonged sleep deprivation and sensory deprivation predispose an individual to depersonalisation.

3.74   Anomia is a contributory factor to suicide.

3.75 Day dreams are more restrained and controlled than night dreams.

3.76 Lithium crosses the blood–brain barrier very readily.

3.77 Graphaesthesia is the inability to recognise individual letters written on a piece of paper despite an ability to read.

3.78 Thought broadcasting is an example of a second-rank symptom of schizophrenia.

3.79 There is a single continuum of disturbed consciousness from full consciousness to full unconsciousness.

3.80 The ego mediates between the id and the super-ego.

3.81 Bioavailability correlates positively with first-pass metabolism.

3.82 Lithium reabsorption occurs at the distal renal tubules.

3.83 There is an established relationship between increased family size and lower intelligence quotient (IQ) when the children are properly assessed.

3.84 The reliability of psychiatric diagnosis is improved by the use of multiaxial classification compared with classification schemes with a single axis.

3.85 The International Statistical Classification of Diseases and Related Health Problems, 10th revision (ICD-10) definition of schizophrenia is narrower and more restrictive than that seen in the Diagnostic and Statistical Manual of Mental Disorders-IV (DSM-IV).

3.86 Schizophrenia is a neurodevelopmental disorder.

3.87 Day dreams often take the form of escapist fantasies.

3.88 First-rank symptoms include second-person auditory hallucinations.

3.89 Cognitive abilities are controlled by lower centres within the midbrain.

3.90 Night-time waking and wandering can cause difficulties for carers of patients with Alzheimer's disease.

3.91 Klein felt that the depressive position predisposed to later depressive disorder.

3.92 Circumstantiality results when thinking becomes non-goal-directed.

3.93 Derealisation is a subjective feeling that you do not exist.

3.94 The Q sort technique involves sorting matchsticks into piles.

3.95 Both tic disorder and hyperkinetic disorders are classified in section F90–98 of the International Statistical Classification of Diseases and Related Health Problems, 10th revision (ICD-10), which covers behavioural and emerging diseases of childhood and adolescence.

3.96 Metonymy is characteristic of schizophrenia.

3.97 The id controls voluntary movement.

3.98 Offer and Offer proposed that adolescence is much more turmoil-filled than is commonly believed.

3.99 Bipolar affective disorders and recurrent depressive disorders are both more common in females than males.

3.100 'Passivity experience' describes the state in chronic schizophrenia in which a patient lacks motivation.

3.101 Biotransformation is synonymous with drug metabolism.

3.102 Flashbacks can be precipitated by a range of sensory stimuli.

3.103 Skinner described attribution theory.

3.104   Haptic hallucinations are perceived deep within the body.

3.105   Kretschmer described pyknic individuals as being solitary.

3.106   Key features of Ganser's syndrome include psychogenic physical symptoms, approximate answers, pseudohallucinations and clear consciousness.

3.107   Munchausen's syndrome is classified with disorders of adult personality and behaviour (F60–69) in the International Statistical Classification of Diseases and Related Health Problems, 10th revision (ICD-10).

3.108   Repeated brief exposure to the conditioned stimulus increases the strength of the conditioned response.

3.109   Dream interpretation aims to discover the latent dream from the manifest dream.

3.110   Emotional lability is characteristic of mania.

3.111   Fortification spectra are experienced during migraines.

3.112   Derealisation usually has an organic cause.

3.113   Stimulus generalisation occurs when a stimulus similar to the conditioned stimulus produces the conditioned response.

3.114   As mood increases, it is described as euthymia, hypomania, mania and hypermania.

3.115   Paranoia involves splitting.

3.116   D2 receptors are only found in postsynaptic locations.

3.117   Intoxication is categorised along with substance abuse problems in section F10–19 in the International Statistical Classification of Diseases and Related Health Problems, 10th revision (ICD-10).

3.118   The critical period hypothesis states that language learning occurs more readily before puberty.

3.119   Reduction and oxidation are involved in the metabolism of drugs.

3.120   Generalised anxiety disorder may involve waking up during nightmares.

3.121   Alcoholic hallucinosis only occurs during periods of abstinence.

3.122   Capgras' syndrome is rarely associated with mental illness.

3.123   The chapter on mental disorder in the International Statistical Classification of Diseases and Related Health Problems, 10th revision (ICD-10) has 24 categories.

3.124   Athetosis is characterised by sudden jerking movements affecting one side of the body which result in a limb being flung away from the trunk.

3.125   The primacy effect states that the first item in a list will be remembered more clearly than other items.

3.126   Allport described four stages of discrimination.

3.127   Eysenck used orthogonal factor analysis.

3.128   A drawing of a family tree can be useful in the recording of a family history.

3.129   Beck described schemata, which he believed were unstable cognitive patterns which interfered with the job of interpreting situations.

3.130   Head injury can lead to generalised intellectual impairment and persistent memory defects, but no personality change.

3.131   Cataplexy, also known as posturing, is a catatonic state involving the maintaining of a posture for long periods of time.

3.132 The term 'latent dream' refers to our memory of the dream when we awake.

3.133 Receptor occupancy is best imaged using magnetic resonance imaging (MRI).

EXTENDED MATCHING ITEMS

3.134   THEME: DRUG–RECEPTOR INTERACTIONS

A α_1-Adrenoceptors
B α_2-Adrenoceptors
C   HI receptors
D   H3 receptors
E   MI muscarinic receptors
F   M2 muscarinic receptors
G   Postsynaptic DI receptors
H   Postsynaptic D2 receptors
I   Presynaptic DI receptors
J   Presynaptic D2 receptors

Choose the receptor type from the list above most associated with each of the following:

1   The site of antipsychotic action of typical antipsychotic drugs.
2   The side-effect of ejaculatory failure occurring with typical antipsychotic drugs.
3   The side-effect of weight gain occurring with typical antipsychotic drugs.

3.135 THEME: NEUROPSYCHOLOGICAL TESTS

A	Benton Test of Visual Recognition
B	Indiana Aphasic Screening Test
C	Memory for Designs Test
D	16-PF questionnaire
E	Randt Memory Scale
F	Rorschach Inkblot Technique
G	WAIS
H	Wisconsin Card Sorting Test
I	WMS

Identify the test from the list above which fits each of the following categories:

1   A projective test
2   A personality test
3   A non-verbal test of cognitive functioning

3.136 THEME: DISORDERS OF THINKING

A	Capgras' syndrome
B	Cotard's syndrome
C	De Clerambault's syndrome
D	Ekbom's syndrome
E	Fregoli's syndrome
F	Ganser's syndrome
G	Gedankenlautwerden
H	Othello's syndrome
I	Sensitive ideas of reference

Choose the most appropriate item from the list above for each of the following:

1   The belief that strangers seen in the street are actually close friends whose appearance has been changed.
2   The belief that radio presenters are talking about you.
3   The belief that one's spouse is unfaithful.

PAPER 3
QUESTIONS

3.137 THEME: MENTAL ILLNESS SECONDARY TO PHYSICAL DISORDERS AND SUBSTANCE USE

A   Both depressive disorder and mania
B   Depressive disorder only
C   Korsakoff's syndrome
D   Mania only
E   Obsessive-compulsive disorder
F   Post-traumatic stress disorder
G   Schizoaffective disorder
H   Schizophrenia
I   Schizophreniform psychosis

Choose the mental illness from the list above most closely associated with each of the following:

1   Cushing's syndrome
2   Pyrexia
3   Corticosteroids

3.138 THEME: PIAGETIAN THEORY

A   Anankastic phase
B   Concrete operational period
C   Formal operational stage
D   Genital stage
E   Identity development period
F   Isolative hibernation
G   Oral stage
H   Preoperational stage
I   Sensorimotor period

Identify the stage from the list above associated with each of the following:

1   The development of circular reactions.
2   The development of hypothetical reasoning ability.
3   The development of a belief in authoritarian morality.

PAPER 3
QUESTIONS

3.139   THEME: PHARMACOKINETICS

A	A steady-state concentration cannot be achieved
B	A steady-state concentration is established in 2–3 half-lives
C	A steady-state is established in one half-life
D	A steady-state is established in 7–10 half-lives
E	Once-daily dosing is required
F	The rate of decay is bi-exponential, suggesting a multicompartmental model
G	The rate of decay is limited by enzyme systems
H	The rate of decay is proportional to the amount of the drug in the body
I	Twice-daily dosing is required

Identify the statement from the list above which is relevant to the following:

1	Zero-order kinetics
2	First-order kinetics
3	Second-order kinetics

3.140   THEME: DISORDERS OF LANGUAGE

A   Agrammatism
B   Alogia
C   Coprolalia
D   Cryptolalia
E   Cryptographia
F   Dysphasia
G   Neologism
H   Paralogia
I   Paraphasia

Identify the descriptive term from the list above for each of the following:

1   Use of a private word in written language.
2   Use of irrelevant words as part of thought disorder.
3   Incorporation of inappropriate sounds into normal words.

3.141   THEME: JUNGIAN THEORY

A	Archetypes
B	The Animus
C	The Collective Unconscious
D	The Great Mother
E	The Hero
F	The Persona
G	The Personal Unconscious
H	The Shadow
I	The Wise Old Man

Identify the Jungian concept from the list above described by each of the following:

1   Unacceptable aspects of the self arising from basic instincts.
2   The masculine prototype.
3   The all-nurturing caretaker.

3.142   THEME: PERSONALITY THEORIES

A	Allport
B	Bandura
C	Cattell
D	Costa and McCrae
E	Eysenck
F	McClelland
G	Rogers
H	Rotter
I	Wilson

Identify the individual from the list above most closely associated with each of the following ideas:

1 Cardinal, central and secondary traits
2 Surface and source traits
3 Theory of locus of control

3.143   THEME: PHARMACOLOGY

A	Acamprosate
B	Chloral hydrate
C	Clozapine
D	Disulfiram
E	Donepezil
F	Flumazenil
G	Methadone
H	Naltrexone
I	Phenobarbital

Identify the substance from the list above which is:

1   A γ-amino butyric acid (GABA) analogue
2   An aldehyde dehydrogenase inhibitor
3   An anticholinesterase

PRACTICE PAPER 3

Answers

INDIVIDUAL STATEMENT QUESTIONS

3.1 **False** – It describes a separate clinical syndrome.
Personalisation is a cognitive error contributing to depression.
A–Z pp 12–14

3.2 **True** – An example is quoted of a weak and passive man who
beats his wife in order to assert himself.
A–Z pp 5–6

3.3 **True** – It is central to the diagnosis.
A–Z p 40

3.4 **True** – For example, dashed lines appear continuous.
A–Z p 176

3.5 **False** – It is an agonist at GABA-B receptors.
Fear p 153

3.6 **False** – It is present on chromosome 21.
A–Z pp 106–10

3.7 **False** – It is pathognomonic of organic disorder.
A–Z p 245

3.8 **True** – They are perceived as scientists, making personal
constructs.
A–Z pp 248–9

3.9 **False** – It is the Schedule for the Assessment of Negative
Symptoms.
Fear p 276

3.10 **False** – Lipid solubility increases speed of absorption.
A–Z p 179

3.11 **False** – It is very soluble in water.
A–Z pp 195–7

3.12 **True** – Although the reasons for this are unclear.
A–Z p 257

3.13 **True** – It is almost always associated with derealisation.
A–Z p 102

3.14 **True** – Although they are repeated in a non-goal-directed way.
Fear pp 97–8

3.15 **True** – They suggest that this is the only reason we can distinguish different emotions.
A–Z p 181

3.16 **True** – Gestalt principles consider the whole to be greater than the sum of its parts and can be used to understand a variety of illusions.
Fear pp 8–11

3.17 **False** – It is found in low concentrations in the cerebellum.
A–Z pp 122–3

3.18 **False** – These are features of a normal grief reaction.
A–Z pp 154–5

3.19 **False** – Negativism is motiveless and results from schizophrenia.
A–Z p 222

3.20 **True** – It occurs when the desired behaviour does not lead to any reward.
A–Z p 192

3.21 **False** – There are no fixed half-lives. The rate of metabolism varies.
Fear p 145

3.22 **True** – So a scared person with arachnophobia might perceive

a crack in a wall as a spider.
A–Z p 176

3.23 **False** – It is an inhibitory neurotransmitter.
A–Z p 151

3.24 **False** – The cerebellum is a dopamine-poor region. D3
receptors are found in the limbic system.
Fear p 155

3.25 **False** – It accounts for over 50% of all cases.
A–Z pp 106–10

3.26 **False** – D1 and D5 receptors are similar.
A–Z pp 122–3

3.27 **False** – Low relative molecular mass increases the rate of
absorption.
A–Z p 179

3.28 **False** – It is the more positive aspect of the ego.
A–Z p 308

3.29 **False** – These are features of a normal grief reaction.
A–Z pp 154–5

3.30 **True** – We realise that the object seems to be getting larger
because it is getting nearer and perceive it as unchanged in
size.
Fear p 10

3.31 **False** – Mutual reciprocity.
A–Z pp 211–12

3.32 **True** – It causes patients to be unaware of which of their
fingers has been touched.
A–Z p 18

3.33 **False** – This is usually the case, but it is not always the case.
Be very wary of questions featuring the word 'always'.
A–Z p 102

3.34   **False** – They are a feature of normal experience.
A–Z p 176

3.35   **True** – An example would be giving the correct answer to the first question asked and the same answer (now wrong) to all subsequent questions.
A–Z p 245

3.36   **False** – There are many contrasting theories.
A–Z pp 21–2

3.37   **True** – It is only 10% for dizygous twins.
A–Z pp 287–91

3.38   **False** – They may be maintained for hours.
Fear pp 97–8

3.39   **True** – Affective symptoms are also common.
A–Z p 99

3.40   **False** – It was used in nomothetic personality theories to identify common personality traits.
A–Z pp 249–51

3.41   **True** – It occurs when the response causes complete escape from the aversive stimulus.
A–Z p 80

3.42   **False** – It means excessive speech and is seen in mania.
A–Z p 199

3.43   **False** – It is strongly associated with clouding of consciousness.
A–Z p 245

3.44   **False** – It is psychoactive and may interact with antidepressants.
Fear p 163

3.45   **False** – It is also seen in Parkinson's disease.
A–Z p 199

3.46 **False** – It is a relative contraindication to intramuscular drug administration.
A–Z p 179

3.47 **True** – Along with Kelly and Freud.
A–Z pp 247–9

3.48 **True** – It involves ever-increasing frequency of utterance.
A–Z p 235

3.49 **False** – They aim to identify common themes that are shared between many individuals.
Fear p 17

3.50 **True** – Typically before the age of 4 years.
A–Z p 114

3.51 **True** – And its potency.
A–Z pp 34–8

3.52 **False** – Diagnostic and Statistical Manual of Mental Disorders.
A–Z p 126

3.53 **False** – This describes retrograde amnesia.
A–Z p 24

3.54 **False** – It can occur in people free from any mental disorder. Be very wary about questions featuring the words 'never' and 'always'.
A–Z p 102

3.55 **False** – Physical examination must be carried out by psychiatrists, as they need to have the relevant expertise and are most fully aware of the relevance of physical disorders to patients' mental states.
Fear p 269

3.56 **True** – They are often perceived as alternating with the background.
A–Z p 146

3.57 **True** – Such as the International Statistical Classification of Diseases and Related Health Problems, 10th revision (ICD-10). A–Z p 105

3.58 **True** – It is a form of perseveration. A–Z p 235

3.59 **False** – Groupthink is almost the opposite. It describes the tendency of groups to disregard minority opinion. A–Z p 157

3.60 **False** – The sensory pathways are intact. A–Z p 17

3.61 **False** – The behaviour is voluntary in operant conditioning. A–Z p 80

3.62 **False** – It is an 'as if' feeling rather than a belief, so it cannot be a delusion. Fear p 99

3.63 **False** – Iconic stores visual information and lasts approximately 0.5 s, whereas echoic memory stores auditory information and lasts approximately 2 s. A–Z p 208, Fear p 13

3.64 **False** – It has no sedative effects at all. A–Z pp 195–7

3.65 **False** – Festinger described cognitive dissonance. A–Z p 119

3.66 **False** – This describes delusions. A–Z pp 175–6

3.67 **True** – They consider individuals to be unique. Fear p 17

3.68 **False** – The logical connections are maintained. A–Z p 74

3.69   **True** – Also in the developing world.
A–Z p 173

3.70   **False** – It usually develops at around 8 months.
A–Z p 211

3.71   **False** – This is not necessarily true. They are often less time-consuming for clinicians than clinician-rated scales.
Fear p 276

3.72   **False** – The optimal delay is only 0.5 s.
A–Z p 80

3.73   **True** – There are many predisposing factors, including mental illness and epilepsy.
A–Z p 102

3.74   **False** – It is the inability to name things, also known as nominal aphasia. Anomie was described by Durkheim as a factor in suicide.
A–Z p 26

3.75   **True** – They are considered to be easier to interpret.
A–Z p 124

3.76   **False** – It is only slightly lipid soluble.
A–Z pp 195–7

3.77   **False** – It is the inability to recognise letters traced on the skin.
A–Z p 154

3.78   **False** – It is a first-rank symptom.
A–Z p 293

3.79   **False** – Some states of altered consciousness would not fit into this continuum. Consider trance, hallucination during drug intoxication or sleep.
A–Z pp 82–3

PAPER 3
ANSWERS

3.80 **True** – It can compromise between the two using dreams or by development of neurotic symptoms or defence mechanisms.
A–Z p 308

3.81 **False** – There is a negative correlation.
Fear p 146

3.82 **False** – At the proximal renal tubules.
A–Z pp 195–7

3.83 **True** – Lower IQ and higher rates of educational and behavioural problems.
A–Z p 144

3.84 **False** – This is not the case.
A–Z p 105

3.85 **False** – The diagnostic criteria in DSM-IV are more restrictive.
A–Z pp 349–50

3.86 **True** – Males are more vulnerable to neurodevelopmental disorders, which may explain why they tend to develop schizophrenia at an earlier age than females.
A–Z pp 287–91

3.87 **True** – They are useful in psychotherapeutic settings.
A–Z p 124

3.88 **False** – They include third-person auditory hallucinations.
A–Z p 293

3.89 **False** – They are controlled by higher centres within the cortex.
A–Z p 76

3.90 **True** – These are features of Alzheimer's disease of moderate severity.
A–Z pp 106–10

3.91 **False** – She stated that it was a normal developmental phase.
A–Z pp 185–6

3.92 **False** – Thinking remains goal-directed, but thoughts are delayed in their progression towards the goal.
A–Z p 74

3.93 **False** – It is the feeling that nothing else exists, apart from the self.
A–Z p 102

3.94 **False** – It involves sorting cards.
A–Z p 248

3.95 **True** – Along with conduct disorder, emotional disorders and disorders of social function.
A–Z pp 349–50

3.96 **True** – It involves using a word similar to the one intended.
A–Z pp 210–11

3.97 **False** – This is the ego.
A–Z p 308

3.98 **False** – They described adolescence as less turbulent than previously found.
A–Z pp 6–8

3.99 **False** – Bipolar affective disorder has equal sex incidence.
A–Z pp 8–12

3.100 **False** – It describes the sensation that one's thoughts, movements or emotions are controlled by outside agencies.
Fear p 99

3.101 **True** – It involves the breakdown of drugs to degradation products, some of which may be active.
A–Z pp 209–10

3.102 **True** – Auditory, visual and olfactory stimuli are commonly involved.
A–Z p 146

PAPER 3
ANSWERS

3.103 **False** – Skinner was involved with operant conditioning. Attribution theory was described by Heider.
A–Z pp 52–3

3.104 **False** – They are superficial. Visceral hallucinations are deep.
A–Z pp 160–1

3.105 **False** – They were described as relaxed and sociable.
A–Z p 188

3.106 **False** – Consciousness is typically clouded.
A–Z p 152

3.107 **True** – With personality disorders and gender disorders.
A–Z pp 349–50

3.108 **True** – This is the process of incubation.
A–Z p 80

3.109 **True** – The aim is to discover the true meaning.
A–Z p 124

3.110 **True** – The mood is rarely consistently elevated.
A–Z p 189

3.111 **True** – They are visual hallucinations perceived as luminous zigzags.
A–Z p 148

3.112 **True** – Often fatigue, but also including temporal lobe epilepsy.
A–Z p 104

3.113 **True** – This is the definition. The conditioned stimulus and conditioned response must be established first for stimulus generalisation to occur.
A–Z p 80

3.114 **False** – Hypermania is not described.

3.115 **True** – Splitting involves the perception of others as either

wholly good or wholly bad. The bad entities are perceived as entirely bad, and paranoia can develop about these entities.
A–Z p 305, Fear p 112

3.116 **False** – They are both pre- and postsynaptic.
Fear p 155

3.117 **False** – It is not classified in the F category along with other mental disorders.
A–Z pp 349–50

3.118 **True** – This is when one's own language is learned.
Fear p 49

3.119 **True** – Also hydrolysis.
A–Z pp 209–10

3.120 **True** – This is a common feature.
A–Z pp 114–15

3.121 **False** – It can occur while drinking.
A–Z p 162

3.122 **False** – it is usually associated with schizophrenia and less often with affective disorder.
A–Z p 70

3.123 **False** – There are 100.
A–Z p 175

3.124 **False** – This is hemiballismus. Athetosis is characterised by slow, writhing movements.
A–Z p 46

3.125 **True** – The recency effect is similar and refers to the final item(s) in a list.

3.126 **False** – There were five – anti-locution, avoidance, discrimination, physical attack and extermination.
A–Z p 105–6

PAPER 3
ANSWERS

3.127 **True** – He was involved with nomothetic personality theories.
A–Z p 142

3.128 **True** – This is often the most appropriate and concise means of recording a family history.
A Guide to Psychiatric Examination p 26

3.129 **False** – Schemata were described by Beck as stable cognitive patterns that formed the basis on which situations could be interpreted.
A–Z pp 12–14

3.130 **False** – It can lead to all of these.
A–Z pp 163–4

3.131 **False** – This describes catalepsy. Cataplexy is sudden generalised weakness occurring in narcolepsy.
A–Z p 70

3.132 **False** – This is the manifest dream. The latent dream is the hidden meaning.
A–Z p 124

3.133 **False** – Positron emission tomography (PET) scans are more useful.
A–Z p 176

EXTENDED MATCHING ITEMS

3.134 THEME: DRUG–RECEPTOR INTERACTIONS

1   **H** – Postsynaptic D2 receptors
2   **A** – α_1-Adrenoceptors
3   **C** – H1 receptors
A–Z pp 34–8

3.135 THEME: NEUROPSYCHOLOGICAL TESTS

1   **F** – Rorschach Inkblot Technique
2   **D** – 16-PF questionnaire
3   **H** – Wisconsin Card Sorting Test

3.136 THEME: DISORDERS OF THINKING

1   **E** – Fregoli's syndrome
2   **I** – Sensitive ideas of reference
3   **H** – Othello's syndrome

3.137 THEME: MENTAL ILLNESS SECONDARY TO PHYSICAL DISORDERS AND SUBSTANCE USE

1   **B** – Depressive disorder only
2   **D** – Mania only
3   **A** – Both depressive disorder and mania

3.138 THEME: PIAGETIAN THEORY

1   **I** – Sensorimotor period
2   **C** – Formal operational stage
3   **H** – Preoperational stage
A–Z pp 356–8

3.139 THEME: PHARMACOKINETICS

1   **G** – The rate of decay is limited by enzyme systems
2   **H** – The rate of decay is proportional to the amount of the drug in the body

3   **F** – The rate of decay is bi-exponential, suggesting a
       multicompartmental model
A–Z pp 251–2

3.140 THEME: DISORDERS OF LANGUAGE

1   **E** – Cryptographia
2   **H** – Paralogia
3   **I** – Paraphasia
A–Z p 88, Fear pp 102–3

3.141 THEME: JUNGIAN THEORY

1   **H** – The Shadow
2   **B** – The Animus
3   **D** – The Great Mother
A–Z pp 182–3

3.142 THEME: PERSONALITY THEORIES

1   **A** – Allport
2   **C** – Cattell
3   **H** – Rotter
Fear pp 17–19

3.143 THEME: PHARMACOLOGY

1   **A** – Acamprosate
2   **D** – Disulfiram
3   **E** – Donepezil

PRACTICE PAPER 4

Time allowed: 90 minutes

INDIVIDUAL STATEMENT QUESTIONS

4.1   Lorenz originally described imprinting in *King Solomon's Ring*.

4.2   Delusions are common in hypomania.

4.3   Adler is associated with masculine protest in women.

4.4   Anna Freud described a number of defence mechanisms.

4.5   Cytochrome p450 enzymes have a role in the oxidation of drugs.

4.6   Cognitive dissonance exists when thoughts, beliefs and attitudes are compatible with one another.

4.7   Jung described the Shadow as the masculine prototype.

4.8   Inability to swallow saliva, and difficulty talking after intramuscular antipsychotic injection probably indicates malingering and can be ignored.

4.9   Likert scales are used to measure verbal fluency.

4.10   The severity of anxiety in depressive disorders does not necessarily correlate with the severity of the depressive disorder.

4.11   Children who adopt the paranoid-schizoid position are more prone to paranoia, but not schizophrenia, in later life.

4.12   The super-ego operates using secondary process thinking.

4.13   The depressive disorder occurring in association with Cushing's disease is often particularly severe.

4.14   Alcohol has a high therapeutic index.

4.15   Semi-structured interviews improve inter-rater reliability of diagnosis for mental illnesses.

4.16   Dichotomous thinking is important in depression and in anorexia nervosa.

4.17   Excessive use of cocaine may lead to morbid jealousy.

4.18   Catalepsy is associated with schizophrenia.

4.19   Language development is well under way long before object permanence is achieved.

4.20   Depressive disorder associated with corticosteroid use is reported to occur in a dose-related manner.

4.21   Humanism is generally positive in its views of the world.

4.22   The semantic differential scale measures affective instability.

4.23   Knight's move thinking preserves the logical associations between thoughts.

4.24   First-pass metabolism is increased by hepatic failure.

4.25   Post-traumatic stress disorder can be assessed using the Impact of Events Scale, which is patient-rated.

4.26   Astereognosia is the inability to determine the source of a sound by hearing alone.

4.27   Jung described an archetype called the Shadow, which was composed of unacceptable parts of one's psyche.

4.28   Type A personalities predispose to ambition and high arousal.

4.29   Klein believed that the anal stage was longer than originally described by Freud.

4.30   The super-ego acts like a conscience, punishing the id.

4.31   Hallucinosis occurs in clouded consciousness.

4.32   Simultaneous conditioning involves the presentation of the unconditioned and conditioned stimuli at the same time, with the conditioned stimulus continuing until after the response occurs.

4.33   Clang associations are a common feature of depressive disorders.

4.34   Asyndesis is characteristic of depression.

4.35   Apperceptive agnosia causes the inability to copy drawings.

4.36   Hallucinosis is the presence of hallucinations associated with clouded consciousness.

4.37   Ganser's syndrome is indicative of malingering.

4.38   Advertence, grimacing and echolalia are associated with schizophrenia.

4.39   Forced grasping is a feature of frontal lobe dysfunction.

4.40   Freud described infants as polymorphously perverse.

4.41   Estimation of time is grossly impaired during periods of hypnosis.

4.42   Persistent delusional disorder rarely lasts longer than 3 months.

4.43   The ego is the most destructive of the three elements of the structural model of the mind.

4.44   Eating a large meal with an oral dose of a drug increases first-pass metabolism.

4.45   Babies with no vision will smile in response to their mothers at the age of 2 months.

PAPER 4 QUESTIONS

4.46 Symptoms in hypochondriacal disorder are usually left-sided.

4.47 Harlow's work supported Bowlby's earlier theory of attachment.

4.48 Beck's cognitive errors in depressive disorder include selective inference and arbitrary abstraction.

4.49 Winnicott felt that babies ought to be considered in isolation.

4.50 Palilalia and logoclonia are examples of perseveration.

4.51 Echopraxia is also known as postural echoing.

4.52 Complications of intramuscular administration of a drug include air embolism and sterile abscess.

4.53 Tyrosine is a precursor of dopamine.

4.54 Redundant clothing a feature of schizophrenia.

4.55 Hallucinations can occur in any modality.

4.56 First-degree relatives of patients with Alzheimer's disease benefit from protection against the same condition.

4.57 Automatic obedience and akinesia are associated with catatonia.

4.58 Perseveration is characteristic of schizophrenia.

4.59 Paraphrenia is classified along with schizophrenia in the F20–29 section of the International Statistical Classification of Diseases and Related Health Problems, 10th revision (ICD-10).

4.60 The volume of distribution of a drug can be calculated accurately with the use of anatomical charts based on height and weight.

4.61 The psychological pillow is a feature of catatonia.

4.62 Modelling can be of use in the treatment of phobias.

4.63 The id operates according to secondary process thinking.

4.64 Jung's Persona equates to the Self.

4.65 The half-life of lithium is 36–48 hours.

4.66 Klein described the super-ego as operating during the first few months of life.

4.67 Automatic obedience is associated with schizophrenia.

4.68 Hallucinations are voluntary.

4.69 Newborn infants can imitate the mouth movements of those around them.

4.70 First-degree relatives of probands with recurrent depressive disorder are at increased risk of unipolar depressive disorder and bipolar affective disorder.

4.71 Hypnotic suggestion can endure beyond the hypnotic state.

4.72 Beck's cognitive triad of depression includes a negative view of self, a negative view of others and other negative cognitions.

4.73 Echopraxia may persist despite instructions to the patient to stop.

4.74 Klein believed that the main defence mechanisms included manic defence and projective identification.

4.75 Persistent delusional disorder is probably a subtype of affective disorder.

4.76 Risk factors for vascular dementia include age, smoking history and intelligence quotient (IQ).

4.77 Tricyclic antidepressants have no effect at D2 receptors.

4.78 Alzheimer's disease is more common in males than females.

4.79 *Mitgehen* involves a lasting change of posture.

4.80 Stupor is associated with both schizophrenia and depressive disorders.

4.81 Akinesia involves reduced motor activity.

4.82 Depersonalisation is much more common in females than in males.

4.83 Schizophrenia has equal sex incidence.

4.84 Administration of sublingual medication, rather than medication that is swallowed, increases first-pass metabolism.

4.85 Stupor involves hyporeflexia.

4.86 Hypnagogic images are seen when waking from deep sleep.

4.87 Erikson described the stage of industry vs confusion.

4.88 Social smiling occurs from 4 weeks.

4.89 Loosening of associations was first described by Bleuler.

4.90 Depersonalisation involves failure of reality testing.

4.91 The primacy effect and the recency effect can both apply to the same list.

4.92 Klein believed that object relations were irrelevant to children and should be disregarded.

4.93 The disorder which is recognised as schizophrenia probably has one cause, which has not been identified.

4.94 Language is lateralised to the right hemisphere in most left-handed people.

4.95   Waxy flexibility is associated with frontal lobe tumours.

4.96   Clozapine is effective in less than 60% of cases of treatment-resistant schizophrenia.

4.97   Carotid bruits are associated with schizophrenia.

4.98   Stupor involves mutism and akinesis.

4.99   Cataplexy often involves physical collapse.

4.100   Dopamine is degraded to dihydroxyphenylacetic acid (DOPAC) and homovanillic acid (HVA).

4.101   Schizophrenia is more common in babies born in autumn, because of a greater rate of early postnatal infection.

4.102   Catalepsy affects females more often than males.

4.103   The process of imprinting is important in the development of attachment in children.

4.104   Diazepam has oxazepam as a metabolite.

4.105   Substituted benzamides include sulpiride.

4.106   Fine tremor may indicate lithium toxicity.

4.107   Down's syndrome is associated with early development of Alzheimer's disease.

4.108   Operant conditioning is involved in learning by trial and error.

4.109   Hysterical disorders can only occur in women.

4.110   Tangentiality is more suggestive of mania than of schizophrenia.

4.111   Apathy and loss of previous interests are early features of Alzheimer's disease.

PAPER 4
QUESTIONS

4.112 All drugs can be given via the intravenous route.

4.113 Ambitendence suggests mental illness or learning difficulties.

4.114 Denial is a defence mechanism seen much more commonly in the developing world than in the developed world.

4.115 The monoamine theory of affective disorder was proposed by Parkes.

4.116 Antipsychotics reduce dopamine production and turnover.

4.117 The fundamental attribution error causes an overestimate in the importance of dispositional factors.

4.118 Attachment patterns destabilise in later childhood.

4.119 Ambitendence is a form of ambivalence.

4.120 There is wide inter-individual variation in the cytochrome p450 system, largely accounted for by genetic factors.

4.121 Stereotypy is a feature of schizophrenia and mental retardation.

4.122 Guilt, and a morbid preoccupation with a sense of worthlessness, indicate the coexistence of a depressive disorder and a grief reaction.

4.123 In post-traumatic stress disorder, it may be difficult to remember the stressful events at will, although they intrude persistently into consciousness at other times.

4.124 Metabotropic receptors have five subunits making up an ion channel.

4.125 Klein believed that the Oedipus complex was experienced during the first year of life, with a longing for the destruction of the father.

4.126 The Structured Clinical Interview for Diagnosis (SCID) is actually not structured.

4.127   Dysphasia occurs earlier than dysphagia in Alzheimer's disease.

4.128   Parotid enlargement occurs in bulimia nervosa but not in anorexia nervosa.

4.129   Second person auditory hallucinations are characteristic of schizophrenia.

4.130   Oblique factor analysis was used by Cattell to investigate traits.

4.131   Haloperidol is a butyrophenone.

4.132   Television influences aggression.

4.133   Lithium is not sedative, depressant or euphoriant.

EXTENDED MATCHING ITEMS

4.134 THEME: DEFENCE MECHANISMS

A	Acting out
B	Denial
C	Displacement
D	Incorporation
E	Introjection
F	Rationalisation
G	Reaction formation
H	Regression
I	Sublimation

Choose the most appropriate defence mechanism from the list above for each of the following clinical scenarios:

1 A 45-year-old man who takes to his bed when unwell and is provided with food, drink and sympathy by his wife.

2 A man hits his wife. He has an unreasonable boss who places excessive demands on him.

3 A woman under great pressure at work who finds training for a half marathon a great way to cope.

4.135   THEME: SCHIZOPHRENIA

A	Bleuler
B	Carl Schneider
C	Crow
D	Freud
E	Klein
F	Kurt Schneider
G	Liddle
H	Murray
I	O'Brien

Choose the figure from the list above who described the following:

1	Fusion
2	The first rank symptoms of schizophrenia
3	The '4 As' of schizophrenia

4.136   THEME: RECEPTOR-MEDIATED EFFECTS OF ANTIDEPRESSANTS

A α_1-Adrenoceptors
B α_2-Adrenoceptors
C γ-Amino butyric acid (GABA)-A
D γ-Amino butyric acid (GABA)-B
E   5-Hydroxytryptamine $(5HT)_2$
F   Ionotropic glutamate receptors
G   Muscarinic acetylcholinergic receptors
H   N-Methyl-D-aspartate (NMDA)
I   Nicotinic acetylcholinergic receptors

Choose the receptor from the list above most closely involved in each of the following effects of antidepressants:

1   Postural hypotension
2   Weight gain
3   Urinary retention

4.137 THEME: CLINICAL FEATURES OF DEMENTING DISORDERS

A   Approximate answers
B   Disorientation in person but not in time
C   Early and marked personality change
D   Life expectancy of 15–20 years from diagnosis
E   Life expectancy of 6 months on diagnosis
F   Onset over 12 hours with complete resolution of symptoms
G   Sleep disturbance with early morning waking
H   Step-wise deterioration and sudden onset
I   Tremor, rigidity and bradykinesia

Choose the most characteristic features from the list above for each of the following:

1   Vascular dementia
2   Lewy body dementia
3   Frontal lobe dementia

PAPER 4
QUESTIONS

4.138 THEME: HISTORY OF PSYCHOPHARMACOLOGY

A	Charpentier
B	Cilag
C	Delay and Deniker
D	Durkheim
E	Janssen
F	Kane
G	Kline
H	Lidz
I	Paraire and Sigwald

Identify the individual(s) from the list above who:

1   First synthesised chlorpromazine
2   Was involved in the reintroduction of clozapine to clinical use
3   Synthesised haloperidol

4.139 THEME: DRUG CLASSIFICATION

A   Chlorpromazine
B   Clozapine
C   Flupentixol
D   Haloperidol
E   Pericyazine
F   Perphenazine
G   Pimozide
H   Pipothiazine
I   Trifluoperazine
J   Zuclopenthixol

Choose the drug from the list above which fits each of the following categories:

1   Aliphatic/aminoalkyl phenothiazine
2   Butyrophenone
3   Diphenylbutylpiperidines

4.140 THEME: EQUIVALENCE IN STAGE THEORIES

A	Autonomy vs shame and doubt
B	Generativity vs stagnation
C	Identity vs confusion
D	Industry vs inferiority
E	Initiative vs guilt
F	Integrity vs despair
G	Intimacy vs isolation
H	Latency vs genital
I	Trust vs mistrust

Identify which of the above stage theories occurs at the same age as the following:

1 Freud's oral stage
2 Freud's anal stage
3 Freud's phallic-Oedipal phase

4.141 THEME: ATTRIBUTION THEORY

A   Correspondent inference
B   Distinctiveness
C   Free choice
D   Fundamental attribution error
E   Naïve psychology
F   Non-common effects
G   Social desirability
H   Theory of causal attributions
I   Theory of mind

Choose the term from the list above described by each of the following:

1   This term was used by Heider to describe the conceptual frameworks used to understand the behaviour of others.
2   This theory proposes that 3 types of evidence must be examined before reaching an accurate conclusion regarding the causes of an event.
3   James and Davis suggested that judgements are made about others' behaviours using this.

4.142 THEME: ANTIPSYCHOTIC–RECEPTOR AFFINITIES

A   Amisulpiride
B   Aripiprazole
C   Chlorpromazine
D   Clozapine
E   Haloperidol
F   Olanzapine
G   Quetiapine
H   Risperidone
I   Zotepine

Choose the antipsychotic from the list above which is characterised by each of the following receptor profiles:

1   High affinity for D4 receptors and low affinity for D2 receptors
2   Partial agonist at D2 receptors
3   Highly D2 selective

4.143 THEME: INTERPERSONAL ATTRACTION

A   Balance theory
B   Effect theory
C   Equity theory
D   Evaluation of alternatives
E   Interdependence theory
F   Investment theory
G   Minimax principle
H   Reinforcement theory
I   Social exchange theory

Choose the theory from the list above which is outlined below:

1   Shared beliefs strengthen bonds between individuals.
2   Costs and benefits are assigned to aspects of friendships.
3   A positive feedback cycle develops after an initial act of
     kindness, increasing mutual attraction.

PAPER 4
QUESTIONS

PRACTICE PAPER 4

Answers

INDIVIDUAL STATEMENT QUESTIONS

4.1 **True** – He was an ethologist.
A–Z p 200

4.2 **False** – They are seen in mania.
A–Z pp 172, 201

4.3 **True** – Women use masculine protest to remedy the inherent
deficiency – their female gender.
A–Z pp 5–6

4.4 **True** – She founded ego psychology.
A–Z p 148

4.5 **True** – This is one of their main functions.
A–Z pp 209–10

4.6 **False** – It exists when there is conflict between these
elements of the psyche.
A–Z p 119

4.7 **False** – The Animus was the masculine prototype.
A–Z pp 182–3

4.8 **False** – It may indicate acute dystonia and represents an
emergency.
A–Z pp 140–2

4.9 **False** – They are used to measure attitudes.
A–Z p 50

4.10 **True** – There may be a correlation, but this is not necessary.
A–Z p 39

4.11 **False** – The paranoid-schizoid position is a normal developmental stage and does not predispose to later disorders.
A–Z pp 185–6

4.12 **True** – This is more sophisticated than primary process thinking.
A–Z p 308

4.13 **True** – It is often severe, with psychotic symptoms.
A–Z p 111

4.14 **False** – It has a relatively low therapeutic index.
Fear p 146

4.15 **True** – They give structure to an interview.
A–Z p 105

4.16 **True** – This is known as 'all or nothing' thinking.
A–Z pp 12–14

4.17 **True** – Although uncommon, this has been reported.
A–Z p 181

4.18 **True** – It is also known as posturing.
A–Z p 70

4.19 **False** – It can only start properly when object permanence is achieved.
A–Z pp 190–1

4.20 **False** – The incidence and severity of the depressive disorder is independent of the dose of the corticosteroid.
A–Z p 103

4.21 **True** – It considers humans to be striving to reach their potential.
A–Z p 167

4.22 **False** – It measures attitudes.
A–Z p 50

4.23   **False** – The logical associations are lost.
A–Z p 187

4.24   **False** – This reduces it.
A–Z p 210

4.25   **True** – This has been widely used.
Fear p 276

4.26   **False** – It is the inability to identify three-dimensional form by touch.
A–Z p 45

4.27   **True** – It is related to the ego and is the opposite of the Persona.
A–Z pp 182–3

4.28   **True** – As described by Friedman and Rosenman.
A–Z p 251

4.29   **False** – She did not describe an anal stage.
A–Z pp 185–6

4.30   **False** – It punishes the ego when it capitulates to the id.
A–Z p 308

4.31   **False** – It occurs in clear consciousness, by definition.
A–Z p 162

4.32   **False** – The conditioned stimulus stops when the response occurs.
A–Z pp 79–80

4.33   **False** – They are seen in mania.
A–Z p 75

4.34   **False** – It is seen in schizophrenia, dementia and confusion and describes fragmentary thoughts.
A–Z p 45

PAPER 4
ANSWERS

4.35 **True** – Shape and colour recognition are also lost.
A–Z p 17

4.36 **False** – It is the presence of hallucinations in clear
consciousness.
A–Z p 161

4.37 **False** – It is a dissociative disorder.
A–Z p 152

4.38 **True** – These are all features of catatonia.
Fear pp 97–8

4.39 **True** – It involves an inability to release objects placed in the
hand.
A–Z p 154

4.40 **True** – He felt that sexual drives were important, from the
first few months of life.
A–Z pp 148–9

4.41 **False** – It is maintained.
A–Z p 171

4.42 **False** – According to the International Statistical Classification
of Diseases and Related Health Problems, 10th revision (ICD-
10), it must last at least 3 months.
A–Z pp 113–14

4.43 **False** – The id is the most destructive.
A–Z p 308

4.44 **False** – It reduces it in most cases.
A–Z p 210

4.45 **True** – This is a reflex.
A–Z p 178

4.46 **True** – The reason for this is unclear.
A–Z pp 171–2

4.47   **False** – Bowlby felt that the provision of food was the most important aspect of attachment. Harlow proved that it was warmth and comfort.
A–Z pp 162–3

4.48   **False** – They include selective abstraction and arbitrary inference.
A–Z pp 12–14

4.49   **False** – He stated that babies cannot be considered in isolation.
A–Z pp 333–4

4.50   **True** – Palilalia is repetition of words, with increasing frequency. Logoclonia is repetition of the final syllable of words.
A–Z p 245

4.51   **True** – They both describe the same phenomenon.
Fear p 97–8

4.52   **True** – Paraldehyde can cause a sterile abscess.
A–Z pp 179–80

4.53   **True** – It is converted to dopamine via DOPA as an intermediate step.
A–Z pp 122–3

4.54   **True** – It involves wearing of several layers of clothes and is associated with catatonia.
Fear pp 97–8

4.55   **True** – Although auditory hallucinations are most common.
A–Z pp 159–61

4.56   **False** – Their relative risk is increased by a factor of 3.
A–Z pp 106–10

4.57   **True** – They are movement disorders of schizophrenia.
Fear pp 97–8

PAPER 4
ANSWERS

4.58 **False** – It is most often seen in dementia.
A–Z p 245

4.59 **False** – It is not included in ICD-10.
A–Z pp 349–50

4.60 **False** – There is no anatomical correlate. The volume of
distribution is determined largely by physiological variables.
Fear p 146

4.61 **True** – It involves holding the head just above an actual pillow
or bed, as if there is an invisible pillow present.
Fear p 98

4.62 **True** – It involves witnessing someone coping well with a
phobic stimulus.
A–Z p 212

4.63 **False** – The primary process thinking which the id uses is
very primitive.
A–Z p 308

4.64 **True** – They are the same thing.
A–Z pp 182–3

4.65 **False** – 12–24 hours.
A–Z pp 195–7

4.66 **True** – She believed that Freud's stages operated much earlier
than he suspected.
A–Z pp 185–6

4.67 **True** – It involves carrying out instructions without question
or delay.
Fear pp 97–8

4.68 **False** – They are involuntary.
A–Z pp 159–60

4.69 **True** – From the time of birth.
A–Z p 177

4.70   **False** – Their risk of bipolar affective disorder is not increased.
A–Z pp 12–14

4.71   **True** – Responses suggested during hypnotic trance can be
elicited after the trance has ended.
A–Z p 171

4.72   **False** – Negative views of self, negative views of current
experience and negative views of the future.
A–Z p 102

4.73   **True** – This is characteristic.
A–Z p 129, Fear p 97

4.74   **False** – Omnipotence, denial and idealism.
A–Z pp 185–6

4.75   **False** – It is a distinct disorder.
A–Z pp 113–14

4.76   **False** – The risk factors are similar to those for cardiovascular
disease and do not include IQ.
A–Z p 99

4.77   **False** – They do bind these receptors and have slight activity
there.
A–Z pp 31–4

4.78   **False** – It is more common in females.
A–Z pp 106–10

4.79   **True** – It is movement in response to light pressure which
stops when the pressure is removed. The posture does not
return to its previous state.
Fear p 98

4.80   **True** – Also mania, epilepsy and dissociative states.
A–Z p 309

4.81   **True** – It is similar to stupor.
Fear p 97

4.82   **False** – There is equal sex incidence.
A–Z p 101

4.83   **True** – Although onset is earlier in males.
A–Z p 285

4.84   **False** – It reduces first-pass metabolism.
Fear p 147

4.85   **False** – Reflexes are normal.
A–Z p 309

4.86   **False** – They are seen on going to sleep.
A–Z p 171

4.87   **False** – Industry vs inferiority.
A–Z p 359

4.88   **True** – It occurs in response to attention.
A–Z p 211

4.89   **True** – It is also known as formal thought disorder.
A–Z p 199

4.90   **False** – Reality testing remains intact. The individual feels *as if* they are unreal, rather than feeling *that* they are unreal.
A–Z p 101

4.91   **True** – This means that the items in the middle are most likely to be forgotten.
Fear p 13

4.92   **False** – She felt they were important.
A–Z pp 185–6

4.93   **False** – The disorder is heterogeneous and different subgroups of schizophrenia probably have different aetiologies.
A–Z pp 287–91

4.94   **False** – It remains in the left hemisphere in 60% of left-handed people.

4.95 **True** – As well as schizophrenia.
A–Z pp 146, 282

4.96 **True** – But it is used because it is more effective than any other drug.
A–Z pp 75–6

4.97 **False** – They are associated with vascular dementia and cerebrovascular accidents.
A Guide to Psychiatric Examination pp 61–3

4.98 **True**
A–Z p 309

4.99 **True** – It is associated with narcolepsy and sufferers often fall down.
A–Z p 70

4.100 **True** – These are the two most significant breakdown products.
A–Z pp 122–3

4.101 **False** – It is more common in late winter/early spring births, probably as a result of prenatal infection.
A–Z pp 287–91

4.102 **True** – The reasons for this are unclear.
A–Z p 70

4.103 **False** – Imprinting does not occur in humans.
A–Z p 177

4.104 **True** – It is an active metabolite.
Fear p 150

4.105 **True** – They are very selective D2 antagonists and therefore have relatively few side effects.
A–Z pp 34–8

4.106 **False** – Coarse tremor indicates toxicity and fine tremor is a characteristic side-effect of lithium at therapeutic doses.
A Guide to Psychiatric Examination pp 61–3

PAPER 4
ANSWERS

4.107 **True** – Because of the amyloid precursor protein gene on chromosome 21.
A–Z pp 106–10

4.108 **True** – Trial and error pairs a voluntary behaviour with a negative or positive response, which is operant conditioning.
A–Z p 80

4.109 **False** – Couvade syndrome is an example of a hysterical disorder that only occurs in males.
A–Z pp 312–13

4.110 **False** – It does not discriminate between the two.
A–Z p 202

4.111 **True** – Initiative is also lost.
A–Z pp 106–10

4.112 **False** – Many drugs are insoluble.
A–Z pp 179–80

4.113 **True** – It is strongly associated with schizophrenia and learning difficulties.
A–Z p 22

4.114 **False** – It is universal.
A–Z pp 185–6

4.115 **False** – It was proposed by Schildkraut in 1965. Parkes described grief reactions.
A–Z pp 12–14

4.116 **False** – They increase both.
A–Z pp 34–8

4.117 **True** – This means that we overestimate the importance of people and their behaviour (dispositional or internal attribution) rather than circumstance or chance (external or situational attribution).
A–Z pp 52–3

4.118 **False** – They are stable.
Fear pp 508–10

4.119 **True** – It is the motor correlate of the mental state of ambivalence.
A–Z p 22

4.120 **True** – An example would be the variations in aldehyde dehydrogenase between white Europeans and some Asians.
Fear pp 149–50

4.121 **True** – Also infantile autism.
A–Z p 306, Fear p 98

4.122 **True** – These are characteristic features.
A–Z pp 155–6

4.123 **True** – This is characteristic of the disorder.
A–Z pp 260–3

4.124 **False** – This describes ionotropic receptors.
Fear pp 151–2

4.125 **True** – She brought Freud's stages forwards to very early life.
A–Z pp 185–6

4.126 **False** – It is structured.
Fear p 275

4.127 **True** – Dysphasia is an early feature.
A–Z pp 106–10

4.128 **False** – It is a feature of both these disorders.
A Guide to Psychiatric Examination pp 61–3

4.129 **False** – Third person auditory hallucinations are characteristic of schizophrenia.
A–Z pp 159–60

4.130 **True** – It is a form of first-order factor analysis.
A–Z pp 249–51

PAPER 4
ANSWERS

4.131 **True** – This class of antipsychotic is potent, with relatively common extrapyramidal side-effects.
A–Z pp 34–8, 162

4.132 **True** – A wide range of media influence aggression, but television is the most powerful.
A–Z p 204

4.133 **True** – This is unusual for a psychotropic drug.
A–Z pp 195–7

EXTENDED MATCHING ITEMS

4.134   THEME: DEFENCE MECHANISMS

1   **H** – Regression
2   **C** – Displacement
3   **I** – Sublimation
A–Z pp 92–3

4.135   THEME: SCHIZOPHRENIA

1   **B** – Carl Schneider
2   **F** – Kurt Schneider
3   **A** – Bleuler

4.136   THEME: RECEPTOR-MEDIATED EFFECTS OF ANTIDEPRESSANTS

1   A – α_1-Adrenoceptors
2   E – 5-Hydroxytryptamine (5HT)$_2$. 5HT$_{1C}$ and H1 receptors are also involved
3   G – Muscarinic acetylcholinergic receptors

4.137   THEME: CLINICAL FEATURES OF DEMENTING DISORDERS

1   **H** – Step-wise deterioration and sudden onset
2   **I** – Tremor, rigidity and bradykinesia
3   **C** – Early and marked personality change

4.138   THEME: HISTORY OF PSYCHOPHARMACOLOGY

1   **A** – Charpentier
2   **F** – Kane
3   **E** – Janssen

4.139   THEME: DRUG CLASSIFICATION

1   **A** – Chlorpromazine. Chlorpromazine, methotrimeprazine and promazine are aliphatic/aminoalkyl phenothiazines

PAPER 4
ANSWERS

2   **D** – Haloperidol. Droperidol, benperidol, etc are all butyrophenones
3   **G** – Pimozide. Pimozide and fluspirilene are both diphenylbutylpiperidines
A–Z pp 34–8

4.140 THEME: EQUIVALENCE IN STAGE THEORIES

1   **I** – Trust vs mistrust
2   **D** – Industry vs inferiority
3   **E** – Initiative vs guilt
A–Z pp 359

4.141 THEME: ATTRIBUTION THEORY

1   **E** – Naïve psychology
2   **A** – Correspondent inference
3   **H** – Theory of causal attributions
Fear pp 32–3

4.142 THEME: ANTIPSYCHOTIC–RECEPTOR AFFINITIES

1   **D** – Clozapine
2   **B** – Aripiprazole
3   **A** – Amisulpiride
Fear pp 166–8

4.143 THEME: INTERPERSONAL ATTRACTION

1   **A** – Balance theory
2   **I** – Social exchange theory
3   **H** – Reinforcement theory
A–Z pp 51–2

PRACTICE PAPER 5

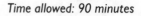

Time allowed: 90 minutes

INDIVIDUAL STATEMENT QUESTIONS

5.1 Adler believed that everyone feels inferior and develops a desire to become superior.

5.2 The Present State Examination (PSE) involves an interviewer feeding results into a computer program to reach a diagnosis.

5.3 Giving approximate answers suggests that the correct answer is known.

5.4 Freud suggested that the anal phase leads to the oral phase.

5.5 Adverse drug interactions can occur when drugs mix in the body and precipitate.

5.6 Klein aimed to cure children of 'psychoses'.

5.7 Hypnagogic auditory hallucinations are strongly suggestive of schizophrenia.

5.8 Ambitendence is pathognomonic of mental illness.

5.9 In cases of secondary depressive disorder, the depressive disorder should be treated vigorously with antidepressants, as the underlying disorder will often resolve.

5.10 Most patients with obsessive-compulsive disorder have motor compulsions.

5.11 Deprivation of attachment can result in a panic-stricken phase.

5.12 γ-Amino butyric acid (GABA) is often found in interneurones.

5.13 Flapping of outstretched hands extended at the wrist may indicated hepatic failure.

5.14 The Q sort technique is primarily a test of frontal lobe function.

5.15 Reaction formation is a defence mechanism that is involved in obsessive-compulsive disorder.

5.16 Antipsychotics increase the seizure threshold.

5.17 Most cases of post-traumatic stress disorder resolve at some point between 6 and 12 months after the original trauma.

5.18 Adler described the 'power of will'.

5.19 The phenomenon of approximate answers is also known as *vorbeigehen*.

5.20 No consistent association has been demonstrated between obstetric difficulties and schizophrenia.

5.21 Disordered self-perception can contribute to the illness in anorexia nervosa.

5.22 Reflexes typically become less pronounced in a patient with hyperthyroidism.

5.23 Muscarinic cholinergic receptors are G-protein linked.

5.24 Social exchange theory suggests that unconscious calculations of the values of friends are performed.

5.25 Block and Haan described anomic extroverts as a type of male adolescent.

5.26 Flashbacks can occur at any time of the day and are unpleasant.

5.27 The active metabolites of citalopram and sertraline have long half-lives.

5.28 Intertwining involving hands and fingers is strongly associated with depressive disorders.

5.29 Ganser's syndrome is dissociative.

5.30 Freud emphasised aggressive rather than sexual drives.

5.31 Alcoholic hallucinosis diminishes in a noisy environment.

5.32 Substance P and vasopressin are found exclusively outside the brain.

5.33 Confusion is suggestive of an organic state.

5.34 Cotard's syndrome is characteristic of schizophrenia.

5.35 Stepwise progression is characteristic of Alzheimer's disease.

5.36 Jung believed that the internal psychic world had mystical elements, in contrast to Freud, who believed it was subject to the laws of determinism.

5.37 Some typical antipsychotics have relatively long half-lives, allowing daily dosage.

5.38 Echolalia involves repetition of another's speech.

5.39 The echoic response involves learning by the child repeating the same word over and over again. It often occurs when the child wakes during the night.

5.40 Episodic memory is responsible for the store of memories of life events.

5.41 Alzheimer's disease is more common than vascular dementia.

5.42 Brief periods of depression are seen in hypomania.

5.43 Physical examination should include repeated measure of blood pressure over 30 minutes to exclude 'white coat hypertension'.

PAPER 5
QUESTIONS

5.44 Field trials were found to be unhelpful in the development of the International Statistical Classification of Diseases and Related Health Problems, 9th revision (ICD-9) and were abandoned for ICD-10.

5.45 Allergic reactions are characterised by immediate onset and dose-related severity.

5.46 Adolescence involves a period of identity diffusion.

5.47 The antidopaminergic effects of antipsychotics on the nigrostriatal pathway cause symptoms of parkinsonism.

5.48 Resistance to obsessions causes a reduction in anxiety in obsessive-compulsive disorder.

5.49 Adler is associated with aggressive strivings.

5.50 Talking past the point is also known as *vorbeireden*.

5.51 Increased concentrations of brain aluminium have been proposed as a protective factor against the development of Alzheimer's disease.

5.52 Extrapyramidal side-effects are caused by the antidopaminergic effects of antipsychotics on the mesolimbic system in the brain.

5.53 Echolalia can occur only when both parties share a common language.

5.54 Sophisticated defence mechanisms include sublimation, rationalisation and undoing.

5.55 Freud described the Oedipal complex in boys as involving fear of castration by the mother.

5.56 A moon-like face is a feature of Addison's disease.

5.57 Zuclopenthixol is a diphenylbutylpiperidine.

5.58 Parenting is influenced by the parent's genetic factors but is independent of the child's genetic factors.

5.59 The super-ego can act as a conscience.

5.60 The defence mechanism of isolation allows very traumatic memories to be recalled with little emotion.

5.61 Global Assessment of Function is classified in the G category of the International Statistical Classification of Diseases and Related Health Problems, 10th revision (ICD-10).

5.62 Victims of major childhood trauma demonstrate unresolved–disorganised attachment in the adult attachment interview.

5.63 Normal grief reactions can include early morning waking.

5.64 Play is always purposeful and leads to achievement of clear goals.

5.65 Gender identity and gender role are always concordant.

5.66 Transitivity tasks relate to comparisons between objects, either real or imagined.

5.67 Profuse sweating may indicate intoxication with sedatives.

5.68 Sublimation is the most sophisticated defence mechanism.

5.69 The HCR-20 system is used to assess risk of self-harm.

5.70 Refractory depressive disorder can occur secondary to influenza.

5.71 Females are more susceptible to acute dystonias than are males.

5.72 *Schnauzkrampf* is a feature of schizophrenia.

5.73 Males are characteristically more aggressive than females.

PAPER 5
QUESTIONS

5.74   Fear of heights is increased when children start to walk.

5.75   Features from more than one Piaget stage can be present at the same time in a child.

5.76   Freud felt that the Oedipal and Electra complexes were resolved by identification with the same-sex parent.

5.77   There is an inverse correlation between the half-life of a drug and its abuse potential.

5.78   Fairbairn and Balint were instrumental in the development of object relations theory.

5.79   Freud's anal stage corresponds to Erikson's stage of autonomy vs shame and doubt.

5.80   Defence mechanisms include acting out, splitting and corporation.

5.81   Smith described social referencing in 1-year-old children.

5.82   Defence mechanisms operate outside conscious awareness.

5.83   Flight of ideas can include punning and rhyming.

5.84   The vulnerability factors identified by Brown and Harris only increase the risk of depression when they coexist with a provoking agent.

5.85   Gilligan's theory emphasises the gender differences in moral judgement.

5.86   Holophrastic speech is over-inclusive in that one word can have many meanings.

5.87   Inheritance of schizophrenia is determined by a single major gene in most cases.

5.88   When their attachment is assessed according to the strange situation experiment, most children are found to have anxious/avoidant attachment.

5.89 Butyrophenone and piperazine phenothiazines are associated with a particularly high risk of extrapyramidal side-effects.

5.90 Transitional objects help with separation-individuation.

5.91 Fertility is reduced in schizophrenia.

5.92 *Mitmachen* involves a lasting change of posture.

5.93 Antipsychotics can cause a dose-related hypothermia or hyperthermia.

5.94 Chloral hydrate is an effective and safe sedative for use in general outpatient settings.

5.95 Hypertelorism is associated with schizophrenia.

5.96 Gender typing starts in infancy.

5.97 Klein placed greater emphasis on aggression than did Freud.

5.98 Cognitive therapy involves modifying behaviour to reduce inappropriate anxiety.

5.99 Adoption studies have shown a much reduced risk of schizophrenia in children born to schizophrenic mothers but who are adopted shortly after birth.

5.100 Freud believed that the genital phase resulted in satisfaction by oral stimulation.

5.101 Although babbling occurs in deaf babies, it does not occur in babies born to deaf-mute parents.

5.102 The relationship between the therapist and the patient is fundamental to the therapeutic process in cognitive behavioural therapy.

PAPER 5
QUESTIONS

5.103 Short-term consequences of deprivation of attachment include protest, despair and privation.

5.104 Approximately 30% of the heritability of schizophrenia is genetic.

5.105 Defence mechanisms are unconscious mental processes.

5.106 Drug interactions can be used to therapeutic advantage.

5.107 Tardive dyskinesia is best treated with discontinuation of an antipsychotic and procyclidine during the withdrawal period.

5.108 Schizophrenia is categorised in the F30–39 section of the International Statistical Classification of Diseases and Related Health Problems, 10th revision (ICD-10).

5.109 According to Klein, the depressive position leads to the paranoid-schizoid position.

5.110 Risk factors for the development of tardive dyskinesia include male gender and old age.

5.111 Attachment behaviour at 3 months is indiscriminate but sustained.

5.112 Benzodiazepines should be the first choice for use in relieving chronic anxiety in patients with a history of drug misuse.

5.113 Regression is a defence mechanism which becomes more active during times of illness or distress.

5.114 Turning against the self is a defence mechanism that can lead to depressive disorders.

5.115 Logoclonia is the repetition of the first syllable of every word.

5.116 Dermatoglyphs are often abnormal in people with schizophrenia.

5.117 Sublimation is a primitive defence mechanism.

5.118   James Bowlby developed attachment theory.

5.119   Understimulation slows language development.

5.120   Monotropic attachment is usually directed to the mother.

5.121   Concepts of conservation develop during the concrete operational period.

5.122   At 9 months, the average infant is more interested in his peers than in his mother.

5.123   The original description of the schizophrenogenic mother has been demonstrated to be inaccurate and misleading.

5.124   Leaders tend to be larger than others but are no different in terms of their health.

5.125   Lanugo hair may indicate a diagnosis of anorexia nervosa.

5.126   The adult attachment interview is used to assess children in order to determine the effects their attachment style will have in later life.

5.127   Szasz believed that schizophrenia had social origins and was not a pathological state.

5.128   Marital skew occurs when there is a dominating father and a passive mother.

5.129   Argyle and Henderson proposed rules of friendship.

5.130   The oropharynx is typically affected in acute dystonia.

5.131   Buspirone is an azapirone.

5.132   Aggression characteristically decreases with age.

5.133   Infectious gaiety is a recognised feature of hypomania.

PAPER 5 QUESTIONS

EXTENDED MATCHING ITEMS

5.134 THEME: FALSE PERCEPTIONS

A	Affect illusion
B	Completion illusion
C	Ecmnesiac hallucinations
D	Extracampine hallucinations
E	Functional hallucinations
F	Haptic hallucinations
G	Imagery
H	Kinaesthetic hallucinations
I	Pareidolic illusion
J	Reflex hallucinations

Identify which of the above most appropriately describes each of the following:

1   A dashed line appears complete when in the periphery of vision.

2   The misperception of a crack in the floor as a snake in a moderately depressed person.

3   Staring hard at weathered bricks in a wall causes them to resemble a face.

5.135   THEME: DRUG CLASSIFICATION

A	Aliphatic/aminoalkyl phenothiazine
B	Benzisoxazole
C	Butyrophenone
D	Dibenzazepine
E	Diphenylbutylpiperidine
F	Piperazine phenothiazine
G	Piperidine phenothiazine
H	Substituted benzamide
I	Thienobenzodiazepine
J	Thioxanthene

Choose the appropriate category from the list above for each of the following drugs:

1   Clozapine
2   Chlorpromazine
3   Amisulpiride

5.136 THEME: DEVELOPMENT OF LANGUAGE

A	Language acquisition device
B	Language arises from children's construction of schemata
C	Language is an illusion
D	Language is externalised thought
E	Language is the result of social pressure from adults
F	Language results from classical conditioning
G	Language results from conflict between the id and the ego
H	Language results from internalisation of social relationships
I	Operant conditioning

Choose the theory from the list above associated with each of the following:

1	Chomsky
2	Skinner
3	Vygotsky

5.137 THEME: SIDE-EFFECTS OF ANTIPSYCHOTICS

A	Acute dystonia
B	Akathisia
C	Convulsions
D	Drowsiness
E	Falls
F	Festinant gait
G	Galactorrhoea
H	Neuroleptic malignant syndrome
I	Parkinsonism

Choose the side-effect from the list above most associated with each of the following:

1   The effects of amisulpiride on the tuberoinfundibular pathway.
2   The action of chlorpromazine on central muscarinic acetylcholinergic pathways.
3   The action of haloperidol on adrenoceptors.

5.138 THEME: PERSONALITY DISORDERS

A	Anankastic
B	Anxious (avoidant)
C	Dependent
D	Dissocial
E	Emotionally unstable – borderline type
F	Emotionally unstable – impulsive type
G	Histrionic
H	Paranoid
I	Schizoid

Choose the type of personality disorder from the list above most associated with each of the following descriptions:

1   A cold, distant and eccentric person.
2   Someone with a selfish disregard for others and a lack of conscience about high-risk behaviour.
3   Extreme shyness and self-doubt.

5.139 THEME: EQUIVALENCE IN STAGE THEORIES

A	Anal expulsive stage
B	Autonomy vs shame and doubt
C	Genital stage
D	Industry vs inferiority
E	Initiative vs guilt
F	Integrity vs despair
G	Oral
H	Paranoid-schizoid position
I	Trust vs mistrust

Choose the stage from the list above which correlates most closely with each of the following:

1   Piaget's preoperational stage
2   Piaget's concrete operational stage
3   Piaget's formal operational stage

5.140 THEME: LANGUAGE DEVELOPMENT

A	Babbling
B	Echoic response
C	Echolalia
D	Holophrastic speech
E	Mand
F	Over-extension
G	Tact
H	Telegraphic speech
I	Transformational grammar

Choose the term from the list above described by the following:

1   Use of the same word, 'mama', to refer to both the mother and the father.
2   Use of a reward for the correct pronunciation of a word.
3   Use of one word to convey a range of meanings beyond the indication of several objects.

5.141   THEME: HISTORY OF PSYCHOPHARMACOLOGY

A	1900s
B	1910s
C	1920s
D	1930s
E	1940s
F	1950s
G	1960s
H	1970s
I	1980s

Choose the decade from the list above which saw each of the following developments in psychopharmacology:

1   The introduction of depot antipsychotics into clinical use.
2   The introduction of selective serotonin reuptake inhibitors into clinical use.
3   The first clinical use of barbiturates.

5.142   THEME: MOTIVATION

A	Actualising tendency
B	Appraisal theory
C	Cognitive dissonance
D	Cognitive labelling theory
E	Drive reduction theory
F	Learned helplessness
G	Need for achievement
H	State–trait model
I	Will to power

Identify the concept from the list above associated with each of the following:

1	Festinger
2	McClelland
3	Canon

5.143 THEME: PARENTS AND CHILDREN

A	Anxious/avoidant
B	Anxious-resistant
C	Authoritarian
D	Authoritative
E	Autocratic
F	Democratic
G	Insecure-disorganised
H	Permissive
I	Secure

Identify the attachment type or parenting style from the list above which is best described as:

1   The type of attachment resulting from a long period of separation from the attachment figure.

2   The type of parenting that places few demands on children and leads to poor social competency.

3   The type of parenting that values children's values and provides definite rules.

PRACTICE PAPER 5

Answers

INDIVIDUAL STATEMENT QUESTIONS

5.1 **True** – Hence the 'will to power'.
A–Z pp 5–6

5.2 **True** – The computer program is called CATEGO.
Fear p 275

5.3 **True** – For example 'How many legs does a dog have?'... '5'.
Also known as *vorbeigehen*.
A–Z p 332

5.4 **False** – The oral phase leads to the anal phase.
A–Z pp 148–9

5.5 **True** – This reaction might be particularly severe.
A–Z pp 274–5

5.6 **True** – Although they are not psychoses as classically
described.
A–Z pp 185–6

5.7 **False** – They are a common normal experience when going
to sleep.
A–Z p 160

5.8 **False** – The only sign that is pathognomonic as far as the
MRCPsych is concerned is perseveration, which is
pathognomonic of an organic disorder.
A–Z p 22

5.9 **False** – The underlying disorder should be investigated and
treated, which will cause the depressive disorder to
resolve.

5.10   **True** – Between 50 and 60%.
        A–Z pp 230–1

5.11   **True** – This was described by Bowlby.
        Fear p 51

5.12   **True** – These are diffusely scattered throughout the brain.
        Fear p 153

5.13   **True** – This is a metabolic flap.
        A Guide to Psychiatric Examination pp 61–3

5.14   **False** – It is a personality assessment.
        A–Z pp 247–9

5.15   **True** – A repressed (and therefore unconscious) wish to
        become dirty is manifest as an over-concern with cleanliness.
        A–Z pp 92–3

5.16   **False** – They all reduce the seizure threshold to a greater or
        lesser extent.
        A–Z pp 34–8

5.17   **False** – Most cases resolve in less than 3 months.
        A–Z pp 260–3

5.18   **False** – He described the 'will to power'.
        A–Z pp 5–6

5.19   **True** – It is a feature of Ganser's syndrome.
        A–Z p 332

5.20   **False** – There is a relationship.
        A–Z pp 287–91

5.21   **True**
        Fear pp 361–2

5.22   **False** – Hyper-reflexia is often seen.
        A Guide to Psychiatric Examination pp 61–3

5.23   **True** – There are many types.
Fear pp 153–4

5.24   **True** – And that friendships are maintained or abandoned on the basis of the results of these calculations.
A–Z pp 51–2

5.25   **True** – They used factor analysis to derive various types of adolescent.
A–Z pp 6–8

5.26   **True** – They are intrusive memories.
A–Z p 146

5.27   **False** – Citalopram has no active metabolites. Sertraline and fluoxetine have.
A–Z p 30

5.28   **False** – It is a feature of catatonia, seen in schizophrenia.
Fear pp 97–8

5.29   **True** – It has been described as a form of pseudodementia.
A–Z p 152

5.30   **False** – He felt that sexual drives were most important.
A–Z pp 148–9

5.31   **False** – The hallucinosis is reduced in a quiet environment.
A–Z p 162

5.32   **False** – They both have roles within the brain.
Fear p 157

5.33   **True** – It is suggestive, but not pathognomonic.
A–Z pp 82–3

5.34   **False** – It is characteristic of depression.
A–Z p 87

5.35   **False** – This is characteristic of vascular dementia.
A–Z p 99

PAPER 5
ANSWERS

5.36   **True** – Jung believed in causality.
A–Z pp 182–3

5.37   **True** – Such as pimozide.
A–Z pp 34–8

5.38   **True** – It is associated with schizophrenia, organic states and
mental retardation.
Fear pp 97–8

5.39   **False** – It is learning by imitation.
Fear p 49

5.40   **True** – Recall demands effort.
A–Z p 207

5.41   **True** – Alzheimer's disease represents over 50% of all cases
of dementing illness.
A–Z pp 106–10

5.42   **True** – These are common.
A–Z p 172

5.43   **False** – This would be excessively time-consuming and should
only be carried out where there is a good indication.
A Guide to Psychiatric Examination pp 61–3

5.44   **False** – Field trials were carried out.
A–Z p 175

5.45   **False** – The onset is delayed and is not dose-related.
A–Z pp 274–5

5.46   **True** – This is a maladaptive time.
A–Z pp 6–8

5.47   **True** – This is the same pathway that is disrupted in
Parkinson's disease.
A–Z pp 34–8

PAPER 5
ANSWERS

PRACTICE PAPERS **161**

5.48   **False** – It causes an increase in anxiety.
A–Z pp 230–1

5.49   **True** – In order to achieve superiority.
A–Z pp 5–6

5.50   **True** – The talker repeatedly gets close to the matter in hand
but fails to address it.
A–Z p 315

5.51   **False** – This has been suggested as a risk factor.
A–Z pp 106–10

5.52   **False** – It is the action on the nigrostriatal pathway which is
responsible.
A–Z pp 140–2

5.53   **False** – The automatic repetition of speech can occur even in
a language the patient does not understand.
A–Z p 129, Fear pp 97–8

5.54   **False** – Sublimation is a sophisticated defence mechanism and
rationalisation is relatively sophisticated, but undoing (also
known as magical undoing) involves the use of superstitious
rituals to minimise conflict and is a primitive defence
mechanism.
A–Z pp 92–3

5.55   **False** – The fear was of castration by the father.
A–Z pp 148–9

5.56   **False** – It is a feature of Cushing's disease.
A Guide to Psychiatric Examination pp 61–3

5.57   **False** – It is a thioxanthene. Diphenylbutylpiperidines include
pimozide and fluspirilene.
A–Z pp 34–8

5.58   **False** – It is dependent on both.
A–Z p 240

5.59 **True** – In contrast to the uncontrolled desires represented by the id.
A–Z p 268

5.60 **True** – They are remembered in isolation from the affect that originally accompanied them.
A–Z pp 92–3

5.61 **False** – It is assessed on axis V of The Diagnostic and Statistical Manual of Mental Disorders-IV (DSM-IV).
Fear p 276

5.62 **True** – This indicates a predisposition to mental disorder in later life.
Fear pp 508–10

5.63 **True** – In stage 2.
A–Z pp 154–5

5.64 **False** – It is often purposeless and does not lead to achievement of defined goals.
A–Z p 257

5.65 **False** – They may be different, resulting in a range of cognitions and behaviours including transvestism. Gender identity is the individual's perception of their own gender. Gender role is composed of the patterns of behaviour that a person adopts in relation to their gender, for example the wearing of male or female clothes.
A–Z p 152

5.66 **True** – They are only solvable with real objects during the concrete operations period.
A–Z pp 253–5

5.67 **False** – It is a good indication of withdrawal from sedatives.
A–Z pp 294–5

5.68 **True** – As described by Anna Freud.
A–Z p 310

5.69 **False** – It assesses risk of violence to others. HCR refers to the historical, clinical and risk management elements of the assessment.
Fear p 276

5.70 **True**
A–Z p 103

5.71 **False** – Male gender is a risk factor.
A–Z pp 140–2

5.72 **True** – It is also known as grimacing.
Fear pp 97–8

5.73 **True** – This is associated with their gender identity.
A–Z p 152

5.74 **True** – This presumably confers a survival advantage.
A–Z pp 144–5

5.75 **True** – This is one of the criticisms of the theory.
A–Z p 255

5.76 **True** – This allowed progression to the latent phase.
A–Z pp 148–9

5.77 **True** – Drugs with short half-lives are more commonly abused.
Fear p 150

5.78 **True** – Along with Winnicott.
Fear p 515

5.79 **True** – The anal expulsive stage precedes the anal retentive stage.
A–Z p 359

5.80 **False** – Incorporation, rather than corporation.
A–Z pp 92–3

5.81 **True** – This involves looking to others for cues when

responding to new stimuli.
A–Z p 302

5.82 **True** – They are unconscious by definition.
Fear pp 111–12

5.83 **True** – This is typical of mania.
A–Z pp 146–7

5.84 **True** – The vulnerability factors include having three or more children under the age of 14 years at home, not working outside the home, the lack of a confiding relationship and loss of one's own mother before the age of 11 years.
A–Z pp 12–14

5.85 **True** – It suggests that males are more concerned with justice and females with care.
Fear p 50

5.86 **True** – 'Horse' might be used to refer to horses, sheep, cows and dogs, for example.
Fear p 49

5.87 **False** – Inheritance is multifactorial, probably involving many genes in combination with environmental factors.
A–Z pp 287–91

5.88 **False** – 70% have secure attachment, with the remainder split between anxious/avoidant and anxious-resistant/ambivalent attachment.

5.89 **True** – These are very potent typical antipsychotic classes.
A–Z pp 140–2

5.90 **True** – They are used by children to reduce anxiety.
A–Z p 227

5.91 **True** – Patients are also more often unmarried.
A–Z p 285

5.92 **False** – *Mitmachen* is movement in response to light pressure

that stops when the pressure stops. The posture returns to its previous state after release of the pressure.
Fear pp 97–8

5.93 **True** – Although this is rare.
A–Z pp 34–8

5.94 **False** – It is potentially harmful and is rarely used.
Fear p 159

5.95 **True** – Along with a wide range of non-specific physical abnormalities.
A–Z pp 287–91

5.96 **True** – This is the process by which individuals form a sense of their own gender. It starts with infant boys and infant girls being treated differently.
A–Z pp 152–3

5.97 **True** – Freud emphasised sexual motives.
A–Z pp 185–6

5.98 **False** – Cognitive therapy addresses cognitions, rather than behaviour.

5.99 **False** – The risk is practically unchanged by adoption.
A–Z pp 287–91

5.100 **False** – This was the oral phase. The genital phase is the adult stage of sexual satisfaction.
A–Z pp 148–9

5.101 **False** – It does.
A–Z p 55

5.102 **False** – It is fundamental to psychodynamic therapy.
Fear pp 511–19

5.103 **False** – They include protest, despair and detachment. Privation is a long-term consequence.
Fear p 51

5.104   **False** – It is closer to 70%.
A–Z pp 287–91

5.105   **True** – They resolve conflict between the id, ego and super-ego.
Fear pp 111–12

5.106   **True** – For example to increase plasma concentrations of one of the drugs involved.
A–Z pp 274–5

5.107   **False** – Anticholinergics such as procyclidine are contraindicated and may exacerbate the condition.
A–Z pp 140–2

5.108   **False** – This is the section relevant to affective disorders. Schizophrenia is found in section F20–29.
A–Z pp 349–50

5.109   **False** – The paranoid-schizoid position leads to the depressive position.
A–Z pp 185–6

5.110   **False** – Females are more at risk. Other risk factors include old age, a history of affective disorder and any diffuse brain injury or disease.
A–Z pp 140–2

5.111   **False** – It is indiscriminate and transient.
Fear pp 508–10

5.112   **False** – They are not recommended for long-term use and should be used with caution.
Fear p 159

5.113   **True** – It involves behaviour characteristic of an earlier stage of development.
A–Z pp 92–3

5.114   **True** – Negative feelings about others lead to negative feelings about oneself.
Fear p 112

5.115 **False** – It is the repetition of the last syllable.
Fear pp 97–8

5.116 **True** – This means finger, palm and sole prints.
A–Z pp 287–91

5.117 **False** – It is a sophisticated defence mechanism.
A–Z pp 92–3

5.118 **False** – It was John Bowlby.
Fear pp 508–10

5.119 **True** – Final language development may be affected as a
result.
A–Z pp 190–1

5.120 **True** – This is the most common form of attachment.
Polytropic attachment (to a range of figures) comes later.
A–Z p 48

5.121 **True** – Between 7 and 12 years of age.
A–Z pp 254–5

5.122 **True** – This is widely reported.
A–Z p 242

5.123 **True** – There is no evidence to support the idea.
A–Z p 150

5.124 **False** – They are also healthier.
A–Z p 192

5.125 **True** – This is a characteristic physical sign.
A Guide to Psychiatric Examination pp 61–3

5.126 **False** – It is used to assess adults.
Fear pp 508–10

5.127 **True** – He felt it was an understandable response to stress.
A–Z p 314

PAPER 5
ANSWERS

5.128 **False** – A dominating mother and a passive father.
A–Z p 203

5.129 **True** – These include giving of emotional support and
repaying of debts and favours.
A–Z pp 149–50

5.130 **True** – The tongue feels large and swallowing can be difficult.
A–Z pp 140–2

5.131 **True** – It is used as an anxiolytic.
Fear p 159

5.132 **True** – Although specific disorders such as dementia may
cause an increase late in life.
A–Z p 17

5.133 **True** – This is rarely sustained.
A–Z p 172

EXTENDED MATCHING ITEMS

5.134 THEME: FALSE PERCEPTIONS

1   **B** – Completion illusions. These increase with inattention
2   **A** – Affect illusion. These are mood-congruent
3   **I** – Pareidolic illusions. These increase with attention
A–Z p 176

5.135 THEME: DRUG CLASSIFICATION

1   **D** – Dibenzazepine
2   **A** – Aliphatic/aminoalkyl phenothiazine
3   **H** – Substituted benzamide
A–Z pp 34–8

5.136 THEME: DEVELOPMENT OF LANGUAGE

1   **A** – Language acquisition device
2   **I** – Operant conditioning
3   **H** – Language results from internalisation of social relationships

5.137 THEME: SIDE-EFFECTS OF ANTIPSYCHOTICS

1   **G** – Galactorrhoea. Gynaecomastia and impotence can also result from hyperprolactinaemia
2   **C** – Convulsions. These pathways also mediate the dose-related pyrexia
3   **E** – Falls. As a result of hypotension

5.138 THEME: PERSONALITY DISORDERS

1   **I** – Schizoid
2   **D** – Dissocial
3   **B** – Anxious (avoidant)
Fear pp 258–60

5.139 THEME: EQUIVALENCE IN STAGE THEORIES

1   **E** – Initiative vs guilt
2   **D** – Industry vs inferiority
3   **C** – Genital stage
A–Z p 359

5.140 THEME: LANGUAGE DEVELOPMENT

1   **F** – Over-extension
2   **G** – Tact
3   **D** – Holophrastic speech
Fear pp 48–9

5.141 THEME: HISTORY OF PSYCHOPHARMACOLOGY

1   **G** – 1960s
2   **I** – 1980s
3   **A** – 1900s
Fear pp 170–1

5.142 THEME: MOTIVATION

1   **C** – Cognitive dissonance
2   **G** – Need for achievement
3   **E** – Drive reduction theory

5.143 THEME: PARENTS AND CHILDREN

1   **A** – Anxious/avoidant
2   **H** – Permissive
3   **D** – Authoritative

PRACTICE PAPER 6

Time allowed: 90 minutes

INDIVIDUAL STATEMENT QUESTIONS

6.1 Digital paraesthesia and subjective difficulty in breathing are features of generalised anxiety disorder.

6.2 Morbid jealousy is associated with paranoia.

6.3 *Mitgehen* is a feature of catatonic schizophrenia.

6.4 Stage theories of development propose that the maturational tasks associated with various stages can be achieved in any order.

6.5 Hallucinations can be eradicated by prolonged, reasoned argument.

6.6 A brain affected by schizophrenia is characteristically lighter than a normal brain.

6.7 The Structured Clinical Interview for Diagnosis (SCID) generates the International Statistical Classification of Diseases and Related Health Problems, 10th revision (ICD-10) diagnoses.

6.8 Higher cortical function characteristically fluctuates in Lewy body dementia.

6.9 At 9 months, infants imitate the behaviour of their peers.

6.10 Klein believed that the Oedipus complex develops much earlier than Freud suggested.

6.11 Athetosis is characterised by slow, writhing, semi-rotatory movements.

6.12 Flight of ideas includes complete loss of logical connections between one thought and another.

6.13   Anhedonia is a characteristic feature of post-traumatic stress disorder.

6.14   Absence of axillary hair may indicate alcohol abuse.

6.15   People with personality type B are never ambitious.

6.16   Antidepressants often have anxiolytic activity.

6.17   Tardive dyskinesia only occurs in patients with schizophrenia.

6.18   Post-traumatic stress disorder develops to the same extent in everyone exposed to a severe trauma. Individual susceptibility does not play a part.

6.19   According to Erikson, the first development task facing a newborn is the establishment of trust vs mistrust.

6.20   There is a relationship between delusional jealousy and excessive alcohol use.

6.21   Muscle tension and tremor can be signs of anger.

6.22   The possibility of formal thought disorder is most appropriately investigated by letting the patient speak at length and without interruption.

6.23   Concomitant administration of fluoxetine and a tricyclic antidepressant will result in an increased concentration of the tricyclic.

6.24   Verbigeration is an example of a stereotypy.

6.25   Gender identity is usually established at some point between 8 and 12 years of age.

6.26   Cotard's syndrome is most common in elderly males.

6.27   The patient should always be allowed to choose where they sit in the interview room. It empowers them.

6.28   Selective serotonin reuptake inhibitors (SSRIs) are more suitable than tricyclic antidepressants for patients with hepatic failure.

6.29   Substitution is an example of a first-rank symptom.

6.30   Catathymic amnesia results from surgery and is characteristically transient.

6.31   Securely attached children enjoy good peer relationships and emotional regulation.

6.32   Dementia can lead to the development of morbid jealousy.

6.33   Some selective serotonin reuptake inhibitors (SSRIs) are associated with a discontinuation syndrome.

6.34   Harlow experimented on primates to demonstrate that food was preferred over warmth.

6.35   Agnosia can occur in any modality.

6.36   Intolerance to a drug is impossible to predict and is dependent solely on the characteristics of the patient, which must be unusual in order for this reaction to occur.

6.37   Eysenck examined personality on two scales, N and O.

6.38   Lilliputian hallucinations are characteristic of schizophrenia.

6.39   Antiepileptics are often enzyme inducers and can act to reduce the concentrations of tricyclic antidepressants, necessitating an increase in the dose of the antidepressant.

6.40   Freud proposed the anal stage, which immediately precedes the oral stage.

6.41   Dreaming is an altered state of consciousness.

6.42   Delayed orgasm is a recognised side-effect of selective serotonin reuptake inhibitors (SSRIs).

PAPER 6 QUESTIONS

6.43   Alcoholic hallucinosis usually involves a single voice.

6.44   Stereotypy is the repetition of goal-directed actions.

6.45   The stage of industry vs inferiority occurs from 6 to 11 years.

6.46   It is most appropriate to start an interview by asking about details of sexual abuse, so that the topic is out of the way.

6.47   Object relations theory proposes that an inanimate object can represent a person in certain circumstances.

6.48   Morbid jealousy only occurs in schizophrenia.

6.49   Conservation of liquid can be demonstrated at a younger age than conservation of volume.

6.50   Nausea and sweating can occur after discontinuation of a tricyclic antidepressant.

6.51   Paroxetine is more sedative than fluoxetine.

6.52   Thought blocking appears similar to an absence seizure in that the patient pauses briefly before resuming their speech.

6.53   If a patient does not mention suicidal thoughts in an interview, it is safe to assume that they have not considered suicide.

6.54   Obsessions occurring as a feature of obsessive-compulsive disorder are recognised as thoughts that are irrational and originate outside one's own mind.

6.55   Essential tremor is an autosomal dominant condition with complete penetrance.

6.56   Allergic reactions involve an interaction between the drug and a protein to form an antibody.

6.57   In the paranoid-schizoid position, the infant perceives other people as complete, understanding that there are both good and bad aspects to others.

6.58 Piaget described circular reactions in the sensorimotor period.

6.59 Socialisation is bidirectional.

6.60 The Q sort technique compares traits between individuals.

6.61 Use of counselling after disasters to prevent post-traumatic stress disorder is based on a broad and well-established evidence base.

6.62 The extent of retrograde amnesia is a good predictor of outcome after head injury.

6.63 *Vorbeireden* is synonymous with *vorbeigehen*.

6.64 The behaviour associated with a psychological pillow is easy to imitate.

6.65 Individuals show less restraint than groups.

6.66 Infants find transitional objects soothing.

6.67 Erikson's stage of industry vs inferiority occurs alongside Freud's latency stage.

6.68 Serotonin and noradrenaline reuptake inhibitors have effects on dopamine reuptake.

6.69 Substitute attachment figures are accepted by 8 months.

6.70 Reflex hallucinations only occur in the presence of a real perceptual stimulus in the same modality; for example, hearing voices only when there is a tap running.

6.71 Carl Schneider described the first-rank symptoms of schizophrenia.

6.72 Jung believed in a collective unconscious, later known as the subjective psyche.

6.73 Normal grief reactions can include a persistent sense of the presence of the deceased.

6.74 A history of mental illness predisposes an individual to development of post-traumatic stress disorder.

6.75 Type II allergic reactions are also known as anaphylactic reactions.

6.76 Episodic and echoic memory are forms of long-term memory.

6.77 Displacement can result in anger being directed towards an innocent object.

6.78 Generalised anxiety features persistent feelings of anxiety all or most of the time, whereas phobic disorders feature anxiety only in response to specific situations.

6.79 Attachment is most strongly directed to the adult who provides the most food.

6.80 Piaget described the stage of intimacy vs isolation.

6.81 Parenting is independent of cultural beliefs about parenting.

6.82 Piaget stated that everyone had reached the formal operational stage by the age of 26 years.

6.83 Sensory memory has a large capacity.

6.84 Negativism involves resistance to all attempts at movement.

6.85 Clinical features of post-traumatic stress disorder include autonomic signs of severe anxiety.

6.86 Babbling is secondary to auditory stimuli and occurs at 6–9 months.

6.87 Duloxetine is a novel selective serotonin reuptake inhibitor.

6.88 Depersonalisation is accompanied by a reduction in anxiety.

6.89   Psychodynamic therapy involves homework and a joint understanding based on scientific experimentation.

6.90   Pseudocyesis is also known as couvade syndrome.

6.91   Following exposure to a traumatic event, the risk of post-traumatic stress disorder is increased if physical injuries were sustained.

6.92   Marital discord in a child's family home predisposes to negative peer interactions.

6.93   Ambitendence involves alternating between opposite movements.

6.94   Mianserin is cardiotoxic and therefore dangerous in overdosage.

6.95   Talking past the point (*vorbeigehen*) can be deliberate.

6.96   Consciousness can be reduced but never increased.

6.97   Plutchik described 10 primary emotions, including acceptance, anger and joy.

6.98   Logoclonia occurs in catatonic schizophrenia.

6.99   Negativism is more suggestive of depressive stupor than of catatonic stupor.

6.100   Attachment behaviour is most prominent between the ages of 3 and 5 years.

6.101   A 14-month-old child's favourite blanket is a good example of a transitional object.

6.102   Behaviour therapy is not useful in treating stereotypy.

6.103   Common side effects of selective serotonin reuptake inhibitors (SSRIs) include diarrhoea, headache and dry mouth.

PAPER 6
QUESTIONS

6.104 Carbamazepine is excreted in significant quantities in breast milk.

6.105 Jasper described five aspects of self-experience.

6.106 Neglect dyslexia includes inattention as a contributory factor.

6.107 Karl Marx believed that the proletariat and the bourgeoisie lived in symbiosis.

6.108 Likert scales assess attitudes by offering statements with five choices.

6.109 The lifetime prevalence and annual prevalence of bipolar affective disorder are approximately equal.

6.110 Denial is prominent in anorexia nervosa.

6.111 Clozapine was introduced and withdrawn, before being reintroduced.

6.112 Emotional lability is a feature of Wernicke's encephalopathy.

6.113 In the Diagnostic and Statistical Manual of Mental Disorders (DSM)-IV, bulimia nervosa is subdivided into the 'purging type' and the 'bingeing type'.

6.114 Kretschmer described picnic, ascetic and diplomatic physiques, each indicating a different type of character.

6.115 Orally administered drugs are prevented from absorption by passive diffusion by gut enzymes.

6.116 Neurotic disorder has equal sex incidence overall.

6.117 Most people with emotionally unstable personality disorder of borderline type have been abused during their childhood.

6.118 Most of the heritability of schizophrenia is accounted for by nurture rather than nature.

6.119 The prognosis of Othello syndrome is good.

6.120 Bandura described triadic reciprocal determinism.

6.121 Only 10% of the population is in social class I.

6.122 De Clerambault's syndrome is usually diagnosed in people of high status.

6.123 It has been suggested that dreams are a way of unlearning useless information.

6.124 Piaget's theory of development proposes that more than one stage of development can exist in an individual.

6.125 Short-term effects of deprivation of attachment include protest, despair and privation.

6.126 Male gender is a risk factor for hypochondriasis.

6.127 Cotard's syndrome is an example of nihilism.

6.128 Idealisation involves splitting.

6.129 After irreversible binding by a monoamine oxidase inhibitor, it takes approximately 2 weeks before monoamine oxidase is resynthesised.

6.130 Social smiling occurs at 4–6 months.

6.131 Benzodiazepines do not induce liver enzymes.

6.132 Anticonvulsants were first used as mood stabilisers in the 1950s.

6.133 Kluver–Bucy syndrome was first described in rats.

EXTENDED MATCHING ITEMS

6.134 THEME: PHARMACOLOGICAL TREATMENT

A	B vitamins
B	Clozapine
C	Electroconvulsive therapy
D	Fluoxetine
E	Intramuscular olanzapine
F	Intramuscular zuclopenthixol decanoate
G	Low-dose risperidone
H	Risperidone
I	Temazepam

Identify the most appropriate treatment from the list above for each of the following:

1   A 45-year-old man with low mood, anhedonia and feelings of worthlessness so severe that he is refusing to eat or drink, saying that he does not deserve to live.

2   An 82-year-old woman with disorientation in time and impaired memory, who is aggressive and physically challenging.

3   A 50-year-old woman with a 5-month history of feelings of low mood, worthlessness and late insomnia.

6.135 THEME: DRUG CLASSIFICATION

A	Clozapine
B	Olanzapine
C	Oxypertine
D	Quetiapine
E	Risperidone
F	Sertindole
G	Sulpiride
H	Tetrabenazine
I	Thioridazine
J	Zotepine

Identify the drug from the list above which is classified as:

1   A benzisoxazole
2   A substituted benzamide
3   A dibenzazepine

6.136   THEME: NEUROTIC, STRESS-RELATED AND SOMATOFORM DISORDERS

A   Acute stress reaction
B   Adjustment disorder
C   Dysmorphophobia
D   Hypochondriacal disorder
E   Malingering
F   Munchausen's syndrome
G   Munchausen's syndrome by proxy
H   Paranoid schizophrenia
I   Persistent delusional disorder
J   Post-traumatic stress disorder

Choose the most likely diagnosis from the list above for each of the following:

1   A man presents to Accident and Emergency reporting extreme pain in his left flank. He gives a history of recurrent renal colic. He smells of alcohol and discussion with the renal physicians reveals that, despite being offered many outpatient appointments, he has never attended.

2   A woman is upset following a rhinoplasty. She feels that her nose is still deformed and demands further surgery.

3   A man believes that he has something very seriously wrong with him. There are no specific symptoms and he is not in pain, but he knows that he has a terrible illness.

6.137 THEME: RECEPTOR AGONISM

A α-Adrenoceptor
B γ-Amino butyric acid (GABA)-A
C D2
D H1
E 5-Hydroxytryptamine (5HT)$_{1A}$
F Kappa
G μ
H Muscarinic acetylcholinergic
I Nicotinic acetylcholinergic

Choose the receptor type from the list above which is the site of agonism of each of the following:

1 Buspirone
2 Bromocriptine
3 Temazepam

6.138   THEME: DISORDERS OF THINKING

A	Capgras' syndrome
B	Cotard's syndrome
C	De Clerambault's syndrome
D	Delusions of reference
E	Ekbom's syndrome
F	Formication
G	Fornication
H	Othello's syndrome
I	Sensitive ideas of reference

Choose the appropriate descriptive term from the list above for each of the following:

1   The belief that there are insects living on one's skin.
2   The belief that a prominent celebrity is in love with you.
3   The belief that one's spouse has been replaced by an impostor.

6.139   THEME: REINFORCEMENT

A   Acquisition
B   Chaining
C   Generalisation
D   Habituation
E   Incubation
F   Law of effect
G   Shaping
H   Stimulus preparedness
I   Trace conditioning

Choose the term from the list above which best describes each of the following:

1   Reinforcement of behaviour, which is changed in small steps, leading to a greater final change in behaviour.
2   The use of reinforcers to teach a task in small stages, which are finally combined to produce the desired behaviour.
3   The stage of conditioning described when the association between the conditioned stimulus and the unconditioned stimulus is being established.

6.140 THEME: DEVELOPMENTAL THEORIES

A   Bandura
B   Bowlby
C   Erikson
D   Freud
E   Gilligan
F   Klein
G   Kohlberg
H   Kohut
I   Piaget

Choose the person from the list above most associated with each of the following:

1   Post-conventional morality – abstract notions of justice and universal ethical principles.
2   Observational learning – as part of social learning theory.
3   Moral relativism – including autonomous morality.

6.141 THEME: GENDER DISTRIBUTION OF PSYCHIATRIC DISORDERS

A	Abnormal grief reaction
B	Alcohol abuse
C	Anankastic personality disorder
D	Anorexia nervosa
E	Deliberate self-harm
F	Depressive disorder
G	Obsessive-compulsive disorder
H	Schizoaffective disorder
I	Specific phobias

Identify the disorder from the above list with the following gender distribution:

1   The disorder with the distribution most skewed towards females.

2   The disorder with the distribution most skewed towards males.

3   The disorder with equal gender distribution.

6.142 THEME: DEVELOPMENTAL STAGE THEORIES

A	Cannon–Bard
B	Erikson
C	Freud
D	James–Lange
E	Klein
F	Kohlberg
G	Piaget
H	Schachter
I	Szasz

Identify the individual(s) from the list above who:

1   Developed a theory of emotion existing only as a function of a somatic state.
2   Developed a stage theory of moral development based on moral dilemmas.
3   Developed a stage theory of development involving schemata.

6.143 THEME: THEORIES AND THEORISTS

A	Klein
B	Freud
C	Kraepelin
D	McClelland
E	Piaget
F	Canon
G	Horney
H	Frankl
I	Beck
J	Jung

Choose the person from the list above most closely associated with each of the following concepts:

1 The Collective Unconscious
2 Dementia praecox
3 The need for achievement

PRACTICE PAPER 6

Answers

INDIVIDUAL STATEMENT QUESTIONS

6.1 **True** – There is no physical reason for breathing difficulties – the sufferer simply feels unable to breathe properly.
A–Z pp 114–15

6.2 **True** – Paranoia centres on the partner.
A–Z p 181

6.3 **True** – It is movement in response to light pressure, which stops when the pressure is removed. The posture does not return to its previous state.
Fear pp 97–8

6.4 **False** – They require the tasks to be completed in a specific order. Failure at one stage does not allow progression to the next stage.
A–Z pp 104–5

6.5 **False** – They are similar to delusions in this respect.
A–Z pp 159–60

6.6 **True** – Lighter, shorter and with internal abnormalities.
A–Z p 291

6.7 **False** – It generates the Diagnostic and Statistical Manual of Mental Disorders (DSM)-IIIR diagnoses.
Fear p 275

6.8 **True** – This is typical.
A–Z pp 97–8

6.9 **True** – They imitate both gesture and laughter.
A–Z p 242

6.10 **True** – She perceived it in the first year of life.
A–Z pp 185–6

6.11 **True** – This is the definition.
A–Z p 46

6.12 **False** – Logical connections are maintained but associations may be loosened.
A–Z pp 146–7

6.13 **True** – It is described along with hyperarousal, intrusive thoughts and images, and avoidance of reminders of the original trauma.
A–Z pp 260–3

6.14 **True** – It is also a finding in anorexia with onset before puberty when pubertal development is subsequently delayed.
A Guide to Psychiatric Examination pp 61–3

6.15 **False** – They may be ambitious but do not tend to appear so 'driven' as those with personality type A.
A–Z p 251

6.16 **True** – More antidepressants are being licensed for this indication.
Fear p 159

6.17 **False** – It can occur after treatment with antipsychotics, antidepressants and in some patients with no mental illness and no exposure to psychotropic medication.
A–Z pp 140–2

6.18 **False** – This is not the case and several important risk factors have been identified, including neuroticism.
A–Z pp 260–3

6.19 **True** – This is accomplished in the first year.
A–Z pp 357–9

6.20 **True** – This is well established.
Fear p 105

PAPER 6
ANSWERS

6.21 **True** – They are a warning sign of possible impending violence during an interview, but there are many other causes.
A Guide to Psychiatric Examination p 100

6.22 **False** – Some specific questions need to be asked, for example to test for concrete thinking.
A Guide to Psychiatric Examination pp 47–8

6.23 **True** – So the dose of the tricyclic may need to be reduced.
A–Z pp 31–4

6.24 **True** – This is the meaningless repetition of sounds.
A–Z p 306

6.25 **False** – It is established by 3–4 years.
A–Z p 152

6.26 **False** – Elderly females.
A–Z p 87

6.27 **False** – It is often important that the interviewer sits nearest to the door, so that they can leave if the patient becomes aggressive.
A Guide to Psychiatric Examination pp 18–19

6.28 **True** – They are much safer in this situation.
A–Z p 30

6.29 **False** – It is a type of thought disorder.
A–Z p 293

6.30 **False** – It involves repression of painful memories.
A–Z pp 23–4

6.31 **True** – They are more confident than insecurely attached children.
A–Z p 307

PAPER 6
ANSWERS

6.32   **True** – This is uncommon.
A–Z p 181

6.33   **True** – Particularly paroxetine.
Fear p 161

6.34   **False** – Harlow demonstrated that warmth was preferred
over food.
Fear pp 50–1

6.35   **True** – Visual agnosia is also known as cortical blindness.
A–Z p 17

6.36   **False** – This describes idiosyncratic reactions. Intolerance is
related to known properties of the drug.
A–Z pp 274–5

6.37   **False** – N and E for neuroticism and extroversion.
A–Z pp 249–51

6.38   **False** – They are characteristic of delirium tremens.
A–Z p 95

6.39   **True** – This is important in clinical practice, where an
antiepileptic may be used to augment the treatment of
depressive disorder.
A–Z p 34

6.40   **False** – The oral stage is the first stage and is followed by the
anal stage.
A–Z pp 355–9

6.41   **True** – Also coma, intoxication and attention.
A–Z pp 82–3

6.42   **True** – Although not common, it is an important reason for
non-compliance.
A–Z p 30

6.43   **True** – This is typical.
A–Z p 162

6.44   **False** – This describes mannerisms. Behaviour in stereotypy is not goal-directed.
A–Z p 306

6.45   **True** – This involves acquisition of important cultural knowledge.
A–Z pp 355–9

6.46   **False** – A rapport needs to be established before this difficult subject can be approached.
A Guide to Psychiatric Examination p 10

6.47   **True** – A blanket can be used for comfort by a child for whom it represents the mother.
Fear p 515

6.48   **False** – It can occur in a range of mental illnesses and personality disorders as well as in an otherwise normal mental state.
A–Z p 181

6.49   **True** – Conservation of liquid is seen at 6–7 years and conservation of volume at 11–12 years.
A–Z pp 254–5

6.50   **True** – Also anxiety, gastrointestinal symptoms and insomnia.
A–Z pp 31–4

6.51   **True** – But sedation is uncommon with either drug.
Fear p 160

6.52   **False** – They are unable to resume their speech, unlike in absence seizures.
A–Z p 322

6.53   **False** – They may be afraid to mention this subject. The psychiatrist must ask specifically about suicidality as it is of crucial importance.
A Guide to Psychiatric Examination pp 67–70

6.54   **False** – They are recognised as one's own thoughts.
A–Z pp 230–1

PAPER 6
ANSWERS

6.55 **False** – Penetrance is incomplete.
Fear p 96

6.56 **False** – They form an antigen.
A–Z pp 274–5

6.57 **False** – Individuals are perceived as part objects. They are split into good and bad objects, which are perceived as different individuals.
A–Z pp 185–6

6.58 **True** – These involve repeated activities, such as shaking a toy.
A–Z p 254

6.59 **True** – This is the process by which one acquires rules from others. They also acquire rules from oneself.
A–Z p 304

6.60 **False** – It only compares traits within individuals.
A–Z pp 247–9

6.61 **False** – The evidence is equivocal at best.
A–Z pp 260–3

6.62 **False** – It correlates poorly with clinical outcome.
A–Z p 24

6.63 **False** – *Vorbeireden* is also known as talking past the point. *Vorbeigehen* is also known as approximate answers.
A–Z p 332

6.64 **False** – It is extremely difficult and uncomfortable for a person with a normal mental state to imitate.
Fear p 98

6.65 **False** – Groups show less restraint.
A–Z p 157

6.66 **True** – They are used for reassurance as the infant undergoes separation-individuation.
A–Z p 227

6.67 **True** – Both occur from 5 or 6 years of age to approximately 11 years of age.
A–Z p 359

6.68 **True** – The clinical relevance of this is unclear.
Fear p 161

6.69 **False** – They are not accepted until 3 years.
Fear pp 508–10

6.70 **False** – This describes functional hallucinations. Reflex hallucinations involve a percept in one modality being perceived in another modality.
A–Z pp 160–1

6.71 **False** – This was Kurt Schneider.
A–Z p 293

6.72 **False** – It was known later as the objective psyche.
A–Z pp 182–3

6.73 **False** – This indicates a pathological grief reaction and is suggestive of unexpected grief syndrome.
A–Z pp 155–7

6.74 **True** – Almost any mental illness is a risk factor.
A–Z pp 260–3

6.75 **False** – Anaphylactic reactions are type I. Type II reactions often present with haematological or liver abnormalities.
A–Z pp 274–5

6.76 **False** – Echoic memory is a type of short-term sensory memory.
A–Z p 208

6.77 **True** – The anger is displaced from its original source onto another person, object or creature.
A–Z pp 92–3

6.78 **True** – This is a key distinguishing feature.
A Guide to Psychiatric Examination p 85

6.79 **False** – It is directed to the adult who provides most comfort and warmth.
A–Z pp 46–7, Fear pp 50-1

6.80 **False** – It was Erikson.
A–Z p 359

6.81 **False** – These are central to parenting behaviour.
A–Z p 240

6.82 **False** – Only a third of people ever achieve it.
A–Z pp 254–5

6.83 **True** – It is also very accurate.
A–Z p 208

6.84 **True** – It is a feature of catatonic schizophrenia.
Fear pp 97–8

6.85 **False** – These indicate an acute stress reaction. Hyperarousal, which is more prolonged but less intense, is a feature of post-traumatic stress disorder.
A–Z pp 260–3

6.86 **False** – It does occur at 6–9 months, but is independent of auditory stimuli and occurs in deaf babies.
A–Z p 55

6.87 **False** – It is a serotonin and noradrenaline reuptake inhibitor, also used for stress incontinence in women.
Fear p 161

6.88 **False** – Anxiety increases.
A–Z pp 101-2

6.89 **False** – This describes cognitive behavioural therapy.
Fear pp 511–12

6.90 **False** – Pseudocyesis is phantom pregnancy. Couvade syndrome is the experiencing of symptoms of pregnancy by a father-to-be.
A–Z pp 312–13

6.91   **True** – This is a recognised risk factor.
A–Z pp 260–3

6.92   **True** – Also juvenile delinquency.
Fear p 56

6.93   **True** – It is seen in schizophrenia and learning difficulties.
A–Z p 22

6.94   **False** – It is non-cardiotoxic and relatively safe in overdosage.
A–Z p 31

6.95   **False** – It can be deliberate, but it is known as *vorbeireden*.
Vorbeigehen is giving approximate answers.
Fear p 98

6.96   **False** – Heightened consciousness is seen in drug intoxication, psychosis and some normal states such as religious experiences.
A–Z p 83

6.97   **False** – He described eight primary emotions, including those mentioned and also anticipation (or expectancy), disgust, fear, sadness and surprise.
A–Z pp 132–3

6.98   **True** – It is the repetition of the last syllable of every word.
A–Z p 199

6.99   **False** – It is more suggestive of catatonic stupor.
A–Z p 309

6.100   **False** – It is most prominent from 6 months to 3 years.
A–Z p 47

6.101   **True** – Transitional objects are first used between 4 and 18 months.
A–Z p 227

6.102   **False** – It does have a role.
A–Z p 306

6.103   **True** – Also vomiting and drowsiness.
A–Z p 30

6.104   **False** – It is not secreted in breast milk.
A–Z p 70

6.105   **False** – Only four were described: awareness of existence
and activity of the self, unity of self, continuity of identity and
boundaries of the self.
Fear p 99

6.106   **True** – Attention will eradicate neglect dyslexia.
A–Z p 127

6.107   **False** – He believed that they would inevitably come into
conflict.
Fear p 85

6.108   **True** – The choices range from 'strongly disagree' to 'strongly
agree'.
A–Z pp 49–51

6.109   **True** – This is attributable to the fact that the disorder lasts
for the whole of one's lifetime, once it develops.
Fear p 233

6.110   **True** – There is denial of the true weight.
A–Z p 100

6.111   **True** – Because of the difficult side-effect profile.
Fear p 170

6.112   **True** – This is characteristic.
A–Z p 189

6.113   **False** – Purging and non-purging. It involves bingeing by
definition.
Fear p 253

6.114   **False** – Pyknic, aesthetic and athletic.
A–Z p 188

6.115 **False** – Passive diffusion occurs across the gut wall.
Fear p 147

6.116 **False** – It is more common in females than in males.
A–Z p 115

6.117 **True** – Over 75%.
Fear p 259

6.118 **False** – Nature (ie genetic factors) accounts for 70% of the heritability. The other 30% is accounted for by nurture (ie environmental factors).
A–Z pp 287–91

6.119 **False** – It is poor, with particular risks for the partner under suspicion.
Fear p 230

6.120 **True** – It is the complex interplay between behaviour, the environment and personal variables.
A–Z p 55

6.121 **False** – Only 5%.
Fear p 86

6.122 **False** – The object of the sufferer's attentions is usually of high status.
A–Z p 91

6.123 **True** – This is the reverse learning theory.
Fear p 23

6.124 **False** – Piaget felt that the individual could only be in one stage at any given time. The fact that this is not the case is a weakness of the theory.
A–Z pp 253–5

6.125 **False** – Protest, despair and detachment. Privation is a long-term effect.
Fear p 51

6.126 **True** – Also low social class and old age.
A–Z pp 171–2

6.127 **True** – It involves the belief that one's body or possessions have ceased to exist.
Fear p 105

6.128 **True** – The good object is then focused on.
A–Z pp 92–3

6.129 **True** – Although this is a continuous process.
Fear p 157

6.130 **False** – 4–6 weeks.
A–Z pp 211–12

6.131 **True** – Unlike many antiepileptics.
A–Z p 59

6.132 **False** – The 1990s.
Fear p 171

6.133 **False** – Monkeys.
A–Z p 314

EXTENDED MATCHING ITEMS

6.134   THEME: PHARMACOLOGICAL TREATMENT

1   **C** – Electroconvulsive therapy
2   **G** – Low-dose risperidone. To control the behavioural symptoms of dementia
3   **D** – Fluoxetine. An antidepressant

6.135   THEME: DRUG CLASSIFICATION

1   **E** – Risperidone
2   **G** – Sulpiride
3   **A** – Clozapine
A–Z p 37

6.136   THEME: NEUROTIC, STRESS-RELATED AND SOMATOFORM DISORDERS

1   **F** – Munchausen's syndrome, also known as factitious disorder
2   **C** – Dysmorphophobia
3   **D** – Hypochondriacal disorder

6.137   THEME: RECEPTOR AGONISM

1   **E** – 5-Hydroxytryptamine $(5HT)_{1A}$
2   **C** – D2
3   **B** – γ-Amino butyric acid (GABA)-A

6.138   THEME: DISORDERS OF THINKING

1   **E** – Ekbom's syndrome. Formication is the sensation of insects; Ekbom's syndrome is the belief
2   **C** – De Clerambault's syndrome
3   **A** – Capgras' syndrome

6.139   THEME: REINFORCEMENT

1   **G** – Shaping
2   **B** – Chaining
3   **A** – Acquisition

PAPER 6
ANSWERS

6.140   THEME: DEVELOPMENTAL THEORIES

1   **G** – Kohlberg
2   **A** – Bandura
3   **I** – Piaget

6.141   THEME: GENDER DISTRIBUTION OF PSYCHIATRIC DISORDERS

1   **D** – Anorexia nervosa
2   **C** – Anankastic personality disorder
3   **G** – Obsessive-compulsive disorder
Fear p 288

6.142   THEME: DEVELOPMENTAL STAGE THEORIES

1   **D** – James–Lange
2   **F** – Kohlberg
3   **G** – Piaget

6.143   THEME: THEORIES AND THEORISTS

1   **J** – Jung
2   **C** – Kraepelin
3   **D** – McClelland

INDEX